CONTENTS

PART I
THE SCIENCE

PART 2:
WHAT COULD GO WRONG IN VAGUS?

PART 3
ACTIVATING YOUR VAGUS NERVE

FOREWORD

I hold a mantra in my heart: The best is yet to come. This statement is particularly true if you've picked up this amazing book, a book that will help you unlock a gift that you have been endowed with from the moment of your conception—vibrant health.

I cannot help but marvel at how amazing the human body is. It is truly the crowning achievement of the universe. At the center of it all is your cosmic interface, the nervous system. The nervous system helps us interact with the beautiful world around us and maintain great health and balance inside of us. It is truly a treasure that we must honor and leverage to live our best life. Our brain connects and regulates our bodily functions through the spinal cord, peripheral nerves, and an information superhighway known as the vagus nerve.

It's no small feat to regulate the function of over 60 trillion cells 24/7/365, but somehow, it's happening at this very moment. Millions of signals are propagating to and from the brain, reaching all the organs and systems in your body, keeping your systems and life in balance. They keep you breathing, digesting, regenerating, repairing, replicating, and regulating. This is all thanks to the vagus nerve.

As we continue to unlock the mysteries of the skies above us and the vastness within us, it's hard not to live in a constant state of awe and wonder of the human potential. This is why I'm so happy that you're devoted to reading this book. I am certain that *Activate Your Vagus Nerve* will move you closer to unleashing your best life!

Dr. Habib has done an excellent job sharing how *you* can claim your most vibrant life by tapping into your inner healing potential. As you navigate the pages of this book, it's vital that you apply the knowledge immediately so you can witness firsthand the powerful capabilities you possess.

Abundant health is not for the taking, it is for the making! *Activate Your Vagus Nerve* will teach you exactly how in a simple, practical, and quantifiable way, but do not let the simplicity of the suggestions fool you. As Leonardo da Vinci said, "Simplicity is the greatest sign of sophistication." I can assure you that there is nothing more sophisticated than your body—which means that there is nothing simpler to take care of. Isn't that what we are all seeking?

The idea that we have to match the body's complexity so we can heal it is not only erroneous but unrealistic. We are witnessing the failings of this paradigm within our allopathic healthcare model. Dr. Bruce Lipton, author of *The Biology of Belief,* refers to this as a "cosmic joke." A true health solution must be a simple one…the laws of the cosmos require it.

Activate your VAGUS NERVE

In these pages you will find powerful, life-changing information. Information that you can immediately apply and share with others. In fact, let me let you in on a little secret. When patients come to The Living Proof Institute (a functional medicine and lifestyle intervention clinic), our primary objective is to apply the information you'll read in this book and get their vagus nerves in working order, so everything else we do together works a hundred times better! We refer to this concept as "autonomic pairing." Patients with healthy nervous systems heal faster and more completely, and require fewer supplements.

You will be amazed at how your sleep quality, digestion, immunity, blood sugar levels, mood, detoxification, and other bodily functions improve without your taking a single pill or potion. Your key to vibrant health is just a few simple steps away. Trust me; my colleagues and I have helped thousands of people by teaching them how to help themselves. Again...no drugs, no pills, no potions, no side effects, and get this, no cost!

In a time where healthcare costs continue to rise, the self-care methods described in this book are of absolutely no cost and only take a few minutes per day. I know it sounds way too good to be true, but it's not. Mark my words!

As you will learn, this knowledge has been applied for thousands of years in all forms of Eastern medicine. You might wonder why no one has ever told you about the simple solutions outlined in this book. The reason might shock you at first but it will become quite clear when you start paying attention to the cues all around you.

You see, the allopathic model of healthcare operates under a paradigm that believes your body makes mistakes, that it does not know how to self-regulate, that there is nothing you can do. Using this framework and convincing others (through marketing) that this is the case, millions of people have been duped into taking prescription medications, mutilating their amazing bodies, and poisoning their mindset. This has resulted in skyrocketing costs, increased dependency on drugs, and failed outcomes. The patient's body is not viewed as a partner on the healing journey but instead as the cause of illness in the first place. Nothing could be further from the truth.

In the vitalistic model of health, we operate under a completely different paradigm. We believe that all your body parts are required, your body can self-regulate, and you can only be healthy when you abide by the laws of nature. We believe that as a human being, you have an innate healing potential that is more powerful than any intervention known to man. We believe that nothing can heal your body better than it can heal itself.

But here is the key...only you can do the work that's outlined in these pages. Only you!

You've been blessed with this amazing life, and this book will help you actually live it.

A healthy functioning and signaling nervous system is of primary importance for those seeking true, life-long health. So, no matter where you are on your health quest, I'm excited for you to apply the knowledge Dr. Habib so graciously shares in the pages that follow.

Activate your vagus, activate your life!

—Sachin Patel, founder of The Living Proof Institute

Activate your VAGUS NERVE

INTRODUCTION

Without your giving it a second thought, your heart will beat 100,000 times today. You will take 23,000 breaths. Your blood will circulate through your body three times per minute, and your liver will continuously cleanse and detoxify that blood. The ever-changing population of bacteria in your gut will work symbiotically with your digestive tract to break down your food and absorb the nutrients required for each of your cells to function. Have you ever wondered how all of this occurs in the absence of conscious control? How do all of these systems work collectively?

The answer is your autonomic nervous system. This system is an evolutionary marvel. It is the part of the nervous system that, put simply, is responsible for the control of bodily functions that are not consciously directed.

Our bodies are designed to live and survive without the need for conscious thought. As humans evolved, our capacity for conscious thought grew exponentially. This was only possible as the systems required for survival became subconsciously regulated, or essentially, automatic. Our forebrains grew and allowed us to think, contemplate, and connect with the world around us. Meanwhile, our brainstem managed to keep us alive and thriving.

The brainstem is the thickest and highest point of the spinal cord. Within the brainstem are many information control centers called nuclei, each with a specific set of functions that it manages and sends or receives signals from.

Some of these systems alert us to internal stressors as well as risks to our survival in the environment. Whether these stressors are due to an infection beginning to grow in our bodies, stressful thoughts about tasks that must be completed, or the physical presence of a tiger in front of us, the automatically controlled functions of this system allow us to survive. These mechanisms are regulated by a branch of the autonomic nervous system called the sympathetic branch (or sympathetic nervous system, for simplicity). The sympathetic nervous system is known to increase heart rate, increase breath rate, decrease depth of breath, shunt blood flow toward muscles in the arms and legs and away from the liver and digestive tract, and dilate the pupils of our eyes. In doing so, this system enables us to fight against stressors or "take flight" and run away from the stressors presenting themselves. When the sympathetic nervous system is active, it is referred to as the "fight-or-flight" state.

In contrast, there is another branch of the autonomic nervous system that allows us to relax and recover from the rigor and tasks of the day. It allows us to remain calm, decrease our heart rate, decrease our breath rate to take deeper, fuller breaths, and shunt blood flow away from the limbs and toward the internal organs, which permits our bodies to recover, remain calm, and even procreate. This branch of the autonomic nervous system is called the parasympathetic branch (for simplicity, the parasympathetic nervous system). When the parasympathetic nervous system is active, it is referred to as the "rest-and-digest" state.

The vast majority of the controls asserted by the parasympathetic nervous system run through a specific pair of nerves in the body—the vagus nerve, which is the focus of this book. This is the only nerve that originates from the brainstem and runs through the entire body. The vagus nerve (actually the vagus nerves, as there are two paired structures, with one present on each side of the body) is responsible for regulating control of the heart, lungs, muscles of the throat and airway, liver, stomach, pancreas, gallbladder, spleen, kidneys, small intestine, and part of the large intestine. How well the vagus nerve functions is a strong determinant of health; vagus nerve dysfunction is highly associated with disease.

We previously believed that nerves had a basic job: to quickly transmit signals from one area to another. We are now learning that the extent of the messages and signals transmitted by the vagus nerve are far vaster and more important than we initially realized; in fact, it is the direct link between the brain and the gut microbiome. The vagus nerve is the single most important communication pathway regarding digestion, nutrient status, and the ever-changing population of bacteria, viruses, yeast, parasites, and worms that live within our digestive tracts.

Balance between the two branches of the autonomic nervous system is crucial to living life fully. Overactivation of one branch can lead to significant loss of function in the opposing branch. Chronic imbalance is what leads us down the path of disease and dysfunction. When stress levels remain too high for too long, the parasympathetic system loses ability to function. Blood flow and function are focused on the sympathetic branch, which means blood flow to the parasympathetic branch will be limited, and thus, function will decrease over time. The opposite is also true, as overactivation of the parasympathetic system can slow your ability to deal with potential stressors and create risks to your survival.

This is a very common issue today, as we live under significant levels of stress and place vast amounts of pressure on ourselves. Our bodies have not yet evolved the ability to distinguish between types of stressors, so mental and emotional stressors elicit the same response as would the presence of a lion, tiger, or bear—something that threatens our survival. This means that we will react identically to imminent physical danger and to our high school teacher yelling "pop quiz" or our boss sternly exclaiming that she needs to see you in her office "immediately."

Under consistent levels of stress, our bodies produce high levels of inflammation and are not given the opportunity to recover and rest, which is required to maintain optimal function. This is why we are breaking down much more easily and commonly than we used to. We are developing autoimmune diseases such as rheumatoid arthritis, Hashimoto's thyroiditis, and multiple sclerosis at higher rates than our medical system can keep up with. We are developing all types of cancers and heart disease and are diagnosed with obesity and diabetes at alarmingly high rates, and collectively, our digestion has never been worse. Given the right opportunity to recover, our bodies can fight back and perform the tasks that our cells were built to perform, allowing us to overcome many of these conditions. The problem is that too many of us are not giving our bodies this opportunity.

We stress ourselves out by eating highly processed foods (which are brought to us by an agricultural system that is more concerned with high yields and convenience than nutritional value) while spending more time indoors, away from nature, and worried about loved ones while forgetting to care for ourselves. Meanwhile, we expect our doctors and health care practitioners to keep up with the demanding pace of change in our lives.

There is a solution to these issues: Take back responsibility for your own health.

Rather than relying on your doctors to manage your health, take back control and use them as a tool to confirm your own theories. Do your own research, learn to manage your own stressors, and figure out the triggers that lead you into a stressed state. Your primary care physicians are a very useful resource, but when you hand over responsibility to a system that is running short on resources and managing hundreds and thousands of patients, you are inevitably setting yourself up for failure.

In this book, I will empower you to take back control of your health. I will help you learn the overlooked root causes of many negative health conditions that your doctor may not yet realize are the true reasons for why your health is so poor. It is likely that your doctor doesn't even realize that there are functional lab tests to help you uncover these blind spots. I will give you practical daily, weekly, and monthly tools that you can use to improve the function of your vagus nerve and parasympathetic nervous system so you can better recover from the stressors of each day.

How This Book Is Organized

This book is organized into three parts.

Part 1 will focus on the science, specifically on the anatomy, neuroanatomy, biochemistry, and specific functions of the vagus nerve and the systems it controls. If you are more of an action taker, this section can be skimmed over. This section is important to read over if you would like to gain a deeper understanding of the specifics of this nerve and its actions.

Part 2 will focus on vagus nerve dysfunction—its signs, symptoms, and root causes, as well as how to measure the function of this nerve with tools you can use each day. This will be an important chapter for those people who are suffering from various health conditions and desire to dig deeper and determine why the problems may be occurring in the first place.

Part 3 will focus on improving and optimizing function. I will outline specific strategies and protocols that industry experts, colleagues, and my patients use when working to improve the function of this nerve to recover and overcome the root causes of their health conditions.

If you are ready to take back responsibility and place your health in your own hands, then buckle up. Let's get right to it!

Activate your VAGUS NERVE

PART 1

THE SCIENCE

CHAPTER 1

WHAT IS THE VAGUS NERVE?

If the human brain were so simple that we could understand it, we would be so simple that we couldn't.

—Emerson W. Pugh

Anatomists were stumped. How could a single nerve beginning in the brainstem be so long and connect to so many different organs? What effects could this nerve possibly employ? With such a vast array of potential functions, what would happen if this nerve was injured or cut?

What Does the Vagus Nerve Do?

The vagus nerve (VN) originates in the brainstem—essentially the trunk of the brain that senses, processes, and regulates the vast majority of the automatic functions of the body. For the most part, we do not have to consciously think about these functions to make them happen. These functions are called autonomic and are regulated by your autonomic nervous system.

Why Is It Called the Vagus Nerve?

Vagus is derived from a Latin word meaning "wandering, rambling, strolling," and to a lesser extent, "uncertain or vague." Due to the vast and non-specific nature of the nerve upon initial examination, the anatomists and researchers wanted a descriptive word that meant exactly this. When they landed on the word vagus, they were in essence calling this nerve "the wanderer."

Some of the functions regulated by the autonomic nervous system include:

- Beating of the heart

- Blinking of eyelids

- Breath rate and depth

- Constriction and dilation of blood vessels

- Detoxification in the liver and kidneys

- Digestion in the digestive tract

- Opening and closing sweat glands

- Producing saliva and tears

What Is the Vagus Nerve?

- Pupil dilation and constriction in eyes

- Sexual arousal

- Urination

Inside the brainstem are various clusters of neuron cell bodies called nuclei. Here, neurons take in information from other cells throughout the body. These nuclei have different functions and are distinguished with Latin-derived names. Nuclei are like a router on a home internet network connection. Some information comes into the router through your cable connection or telephone line, the information is processed in the router, and other information is then sent out from the router to your computer, television, and any other electronics that are connected to your network.

There are two main types of neurons, and they send information in one of two directions. The first are afferent neurons, which receive information about what is taking place in and around the body. Afferent neurons take information from the body toward the brain, called afferent information. The second are called efferent neurons, which send out information with regulatory or motor effects (called efferent information) to various organs and structures throughout the body, so efferent information is carried from the brain, toward the body.

The vagus nerve is connected to four different nuclei within the brainstem. Eighty percent of the information transmitted by the VN is afferent information, meaning that the most common direction that information flows in the VN is from the organs of the body to the brain. The remaining 20 percent of the neurons in the VN have an efferent signal, from the brain to the body, leading to specific functions taking place in each cell and organ. It's intriguing to learn that most medical students are shocked at the fact that only 20 percent of the VN's function is efferent, as it has so many efferent effects on the organs—just imagine then the amount of information that this nerve relays back to the brain, more than four times as much as the information it relays away from it.

Like the wires of your home network connection, the bundles of neurons within your nerves send information along their length using electrical signals, which, upon reaching the end of the nerve, lead to the release of a chemical signal called a neurotransmitter. These neurotransmitters will bind to receptors on the receiving cells, leading to an effect in the cells at the end of the connection. The major neurotransmitter utilized by the VN is called acetylcholine (ACh for short), which has a major anti-inflammatory effect in the body.

Managing the inflammatory system is one of the most important functions of the VN; it is the major inflammatory control system in the body and has far-reaching effects on your personal state of health and disease. Many of the health conditions that my patients suffer from are due to high levels of inflammation in certain organs and systems, from the digestive tract to the liver and even the brain.

Inflammation is an important response within the body to keep us safe from bacterial and viral invaders, physical trauma, and other things that should optimally not enter the body. When inflammation levels are not kept in check and become chronic, the effects can be wide-ranging and lead to many different health conditions. Some common conditions correlated to high inflammation levels include:

- Alzheimer's disease

- Arthritis

- Asthma

- Cancer

- Crohn's disease

- Diabetes

- Heart and cardiovascular disease

- High blood pressure

- High cholesterol

- Postural orthostatic tachycardia syndrome (POTS)

- Ulcerative colitis

- As well as any condition that ends in the suffix –itis

Most of the organs affected in these conditions are innervated (or connected) by the VN. Thus, it is not just possible but highly likely that the VN is working suboptimally and not having its anti-inflammatory effect on these organs, leading to chronic inflammation and disease.

It's important to remember that these conditions do not occur in isolation and if one of these conditions is present, another is likely to be taking place. The same signals are sent through the vagus nerve to and from nearly each internal organ, so if inflammation levels are not controlled in one organ, the same is likely occurring in other areas.

Activate your VAGUS NERVE

CHAPTER 2

WHERE IS THE VAGUS NERVE LOCATED?

The vagus nerve is the longest nerve in the body. Without getting too technical, I want to explain where the nerve starts and how it courses and reaches the organs that it innervates and sends information to and from. Let's follow its course through the body.

Brainstem Connections

The neurons that form the vagus nerve begin in the brainstem, stemming from four different nuclei. These nuclei consist of the dorsal motor nucleus, nucleus solitarius (solitary nucleus), spinal trigeminal nucleus, and nucleus ambiguus. Each of these nuclei control specific component fibers of the nerve.

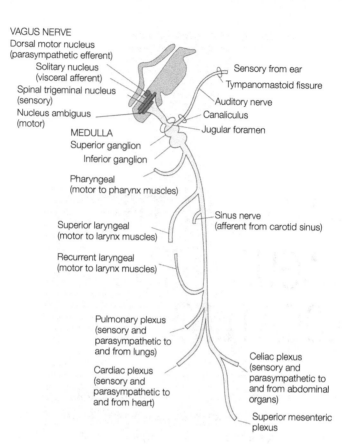

VAGUS NERVE
Dorsal motor nucleus
(parasympathetic efferent)
Solitary nucleus
(visceral afferent)
Spinal trigeminal nucleus
(sensory)
Nucleus ambiguus
(motor)
MEDULLA
Superior ganglion
Inferior ganglion
Pharyngeal
(motor to pharynx muscles)
Superior laryngeal
(motor to larynx muscles)
Recurrent laryngeal
(motor to larynx muscles)
Pulmonary plexus
(sensory and
parasympathetic to
and from lungs)
Cardiac plexus
(sensory and
parasympathetic to
and from heart)

Sensory from ear
Tympanomastoid fissure
Auditory nerve
Canaliculus
Jugular foramen
Sinus nerve
(afferent from carotid sinus)
Celiac plexus
(sensory and
parasympathetic to
and from abdominal
organs)
Superior mesenteric
plexus

Sensory neurons bring signals from the skin that the vagus nerve innervates to the spinal trigeminal nucleus. This includes a specific section of skin of the ear, which is important when it comes to activating the vagus nerve using acupuncture treatment and will be discussed in later chapters. Signals from the internal organs of the body are brought to the solitary nucleus via the vagus nerve and moved up into the brain for further processing. These signals include those from the stomach, intestinal tract, lungs, heart, liver, gallbladder, pancreas, and spleen. We are also able to send direct signals to these organs through the vagus nerve using parasympathetic

Activate your VAGUS NERVE

fibers that originate in the dorsal motor nucleus. These signals help to calm and regulate the function of the heart and lungs and increase the action of the gut and intestinal tract, liver, pancreas, gallbladder, and spleen.

The final nucleus that contributes fibers to the VN is the nucleus ambiguus. This nucleus sends out neurons that have a motor function, specifically working to control the majority of muscles present in the throat and upper airway. These muscles are responsible for keeping the airway open and producing sound using the vocal cords, thus creating your voice.

The right and left vagus are the only nerves in the body with four different functions and four distinct nuclei that specifically contribute component fibers. Most other nerves in the body carry simple sensory information from the skin and motor signals for movement to the muscles. This simple distinction should make you aware of how important the vagus nerve truly is and the wide extent of its function.

Now, let's follow the path of the nerves from the brainstem downward into the neck, thorax (chest area), and abdomen (belly area).

Into the Neck

From the area of the brainstem known as the medulla oblongata, fibers of the left and right vagus nerves extend into the cranial cavity (the inside of the skull) and converge to form what we call the vagus nerve. The nerve then passes out of the skull through an opening called the jugular foramen. This opening is a large space for the nerve and other blood vessels to pass between the neck and the skull. Once the VN exits the skull, it enters the upper neck area just behind the ear, between the internal jugular vein and internal carotid artery. These blood vessels are the direct lines of blood to and from the brain and are extremely important in keeping us alive.

Being in such close proximity to these specific blood vessels is a clue to just how important the vagus nerve is, as physical damage to any of these three structures can cause irreparable damage. In the case of the blood vessels, damage can lead directly to death while damage to the nerve will lead to a complete lack of function in many organs of the body.

Immediately after the vagus passes through the jugular foramen is a thickening of the nerve called the superior ganglion (or jugular ganglion). A ganglion is a thickening of a nerve formed by a collection of sensory neuron cell bodies located in very close proximity to one another. The cell bodies of the sensory nerves congregate in this ganglion and then reform into the thinner nerve section, which gives rise to the first branch of the vagus nerve.

The first branch of the VN is called the auricular branch. The auricular branch passes back into the skull through an opening called the mastoid canaliculus and toward the ear through another hole of the skull called the tympanomastoid fissure. The nerve extends toward the skin of each ear. This branch senses touch, temperature, and wetness on the skin of the ear; specifically, the external canal, tragus, and auricle. It is the main target for activation treatment of VN dysfunction using auricular acupuncture (acupuncture points in the ear), which we will discuss in later chapters.

As the nerve begins passing downward (or inferiorly, using anatomical language) from the superior ganglion, the VN thickens once again to form the inferior ganglion, also known as the nodose ganglion. This ganglion houses the cell bodies of the neurons that are involved in bringing information from the internal organs. The nerve then thins out again and immediately enters a passageway created by a thickening of connective tissue called the carotid sheath. Along with the internal carotid artery and internal jugular vein, the vagus nerve is given extra soft tissue protection as it passes down through the neck.

Within the carotid sheath, the vagus nerve gives off its next branch: the pharyngeal branch. The pharyngeal branch has neurons from the vagus nerve but also carries some contributing neurons from the ninth and eleventh cranial nerves (glossopharyngeal and accessory nerves). Once these neurons converge, they will pass toward the midline of the body until they reach the upper part of the throat, called the pharynx. In the pharynx, the vagus nerve relays motor signals to multiple muscles that are involved in the swallowing reflex, managing the opening and closing of the upper airway, and maintaining the gag reflex.

As the vagus nerve descends the sides of the neck within the carotid sheath, it gives rise to the third branch, known as the superior laryngeal nerve. This nerve branches from the VN quite soon after the pharyngeal branch, and supplies motor signaling to the muscles of the larynx above the vocal cords, specifically the muscles that control the pitch of your voice.

As the VN courses down through the carotid sheath, it gives rise to the cervical cardiac branches, which are two of the three branches that innervate the heart. The third branch, the thoracic cardiac branch, arises soon after leaving the carotid sheath in the chest (thorax) area. These branches intermingle with nerves of the sympathetic nervous system and form the cardiac plexus (a plexus, pluralized as plexi, is a collection of intermingling nerve fibers of different branches and different origin nerves that courses toward a specific location). We have two cardiac plexi: one in front of the aorta called the superficial cardiac plexus, and one behind the arch of the aorta called the deep cardiac plexus. (The aorta is the primary blood vessel, which carries blood from the heart to the rest of the body.)

Some fibers of the cardiac plexi extend toward the sinoatrial (SA) node of the heart, while others will extend toward the atrioventricular (AV) node. We will discuss the function of these nerves on the heart in the next chapter. For now, the most important thing to remember is that these fibers control the rate of electrical activity that pumps your heart.

Into the Thorax

After the nerve exits the bottom of the sheath, it courses downward into the thorax, behind the first and second ribs, and in front of the larger blood vessels that extend from the heart.

The left vagus nerve passes in front of (anterior to) the arch of the aorta and then sends off its fourth branch—the recurrent laryngeal nerve. On the opposite side of the body, the right vagus nerve follows a similar path; however, it passes in front of the right subclavian artery and then sends off its fourth branch, the right side recurrent laryngeal nerve.

Both recurrent laryngeal nerves follow a similar path, but on opposite sides of the body. These are the only branches of the nerve that turn and course upward toward the neck again. They carry motor signals from the brainstem to each of the

Activate your VAGUS NERVE

larynx muscles below the vocal cords, which are important for the production of vocal sounds, based on tensioning and loosening of the vocal cords. We will discuss more about how we can use these specific branches to help improve the vagus nerve if it is functioning suboptimally.

Once the nerves reach the level of the aorta, each one of the vagus nerves sends off branches to the next pair of organs, the lungs. The left vagus nerve sends a pulmonary branch to the anterior pulmonary plexus and the right vagus nerve sends a pulmonary branch to the posterior pulmonary plexus. These nerve branches mix with sympathetic neurons, reorganize, then travel to each side to innervate the lungs. These branches go to the bronchi and larger branches of the lungs to open and close them according to the need of the body based on each situation.

One organ in the thorax that the vagus nerve innervates is often highly overlooked or forgotten about: the thymus. The thymus is an extremely important organ of the immune system. It is located in the mediastinum of the chest, in front of the heart but behind the sternum. A branch of the vagus makes its way to this nerve to send signals to and from the thymus. The thymus forms early in our development and is the major source of training for and growth of our white blood cells. The reason this organ is so easily forgotten is that over time, it shrinks and is replaced by fat tissue. This process begins during puberty and can continue for many years into early adulthood. I like to think of the thymus as a school for new immune cells, and as the school gets old and deteriorates, the training that the white blood cells go through decreases in quality. We will discuss the role of the thymus in much greater detail in later chapters.

Into the Abdomen

The final section that the vagus nerve innervates is the organs of the abdomen. These organs are important for digestion, controlling the immune system, and ensuring that the blood reaching the rest of our cells does not contain toxins that can negatively affect cell health.

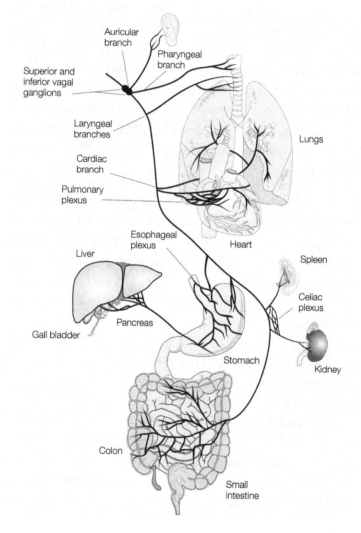

The first abdominal branch of the vagus nerve goes to the stomach. When our body is in the rest-and-digest state, the fibers of the vagus nerve stimulate stomach muscles to function. They send signals to the parietal cells to produce and secrete hydrochloric acid (HCl), the chief cells to produce and secrete the digestive enzymes pepsin and gastrin, and the smooth muscle cells of the stomach to physically churn and push the food in our stomach into the next section of the digestive tract, the small intestine.

If the vagus nerve is damaged and not sending these important signals to the cells of the stomach, it will lead to issues such as hypochlorhydria, or low stomach acid, which is a major root cause of many health conditions. Sufficiently low pH (high acid) is needed for activating digestive enzymes and breaking down food. The optimal range of stomach pH should be around 3.0 in the stomach, while nothing above 5.0 will be strong enough to activate pepsin and gastrin. Low stomach acid makes food breakdown less optimal. Higher pH in the stomach can also allow unwanted bacteria, viruses, and parasites to make their way into the intestines and wreak havoc on your digestive tract.

The second abdominal branch of the vagus goes to the liver. Interestingly, these branches are strongly linked to the sensation of hunger and desire for certain types of nutrients. The food that we eat initially enters the stomach to be broken down. It then enters the small intestine, where most of our macronutrients (fats, carbohydrates, and amino acids from protein) are absorbed into the bloodstream. These nutrients then flow into the liver via the portal vein for filtration, processing, and sending signals back up to the brain.

From the liver, the vagus relays information to the brain regarding blood sugar balance, intake of fats, and overall liver function. The vagus nerve can also relay information regarding the amount of bile necessary to help in the digestion of fats. The liver has many functions that require vagus input, including and certainly not limited to production of bile and bile salts (the active component of bile), which are then sent to the gallbladder for storage; balancing the blood sugar through production of glucose; managing hunger and satiety through the measurement of fat intake; filtration of blood in the portal vein, which brings all nutrients and toxins from the gut; and phase 1 and phase 2 of detoxification processes for fat-soluble hormones, neurotransmitters, and toxins from the body. The liver is very important to our overall well-being and the vagus innervation is strongly associated with maintaining this balance.

Intimately connected to the liver is the gallbladder. Often overlooked by the medical system, the gallbladder is important for optimal function of our bodies. When the liver creates bile and bile salts, they are sent to the gallbladder for storage in preparation for the next meal. When the next meal occurs, the gallbladder pumps bile into the duodenum (the first part of the small intestine) to help bring fats into the bloodstream. The pump of the gallbladder is mediated by the vagus nerve. From the liver, the vagus branches off to send signals to the gallbladder, activating the smooth muscle cells in its walls to pump bile into the digestive tract. This happens in response to a meal that the taste buds (sensory receptors on the tongue) determined contained fat, which should be digested once it reaches the small intestine.

Activate your VAGUS NERVE

The next branch of the vagus is directed toward the pancreas. Your pancreas is one of the most important glands in your body, with both an exocrine and endocrine component. The endocrine pancreas produces and secretes insulin and glucagon directly into the bloodstream to balance glucose levels in the blood (blood sugar). The exocrine pancreas produces and secretes digestive enzymes through a duct directly into the small intestine. The three most notable digestive enzymes produced by the pancreas are protease, which breaks down proteins into their component amino acids; lipase, which breaks down fats from their component triglycerides into free fatty acids and cholesterol; and amylase, which breaks down carbohydrates into simpler sugars.

Vagus innervation sends signals from the pancreas back to the brainstem, relaying information regarding exocrine and endocrine cell status. It also relays information from the brainstem back to the organ regarding food intake and which enzymes are required for production and release into the bloodstream and digestive tract. Vagus innervation is essential for relaying this information because a lack of signaling will alter the release of digestive enzymes, reducing the effectiveness of the digestive process.

Once the vagus nerve courses past the stomach, it forms the celiac plexus, which is a network formed between lumbar sympathetic nerves and the parasympathetic fibers of the vagus. This network sends branches to the remaining organs in the abdomen.

The first organ innervated after the celiac plexus is the spleen. The spleen is located on the left side of your body, below the left lung, opposite the liver. Its function is to monitor the bloodstream and activate or deactivate cells of the immune system based on what it senses. Early in our lives, both the spleen and the thymus manage immune cell function, but later in life once the thymus has disappeared, this system is managed by just the spleen.

The spleen receives messages from the sympathetic branches to activate the inflammatory pathways, which turn on in response to physical and biochemical trauma or damage. The parasympathetic branches send signals to halt the inflammation processes. The vagus nerve modulates a system called the cholinergic anti-inflammatory pathway, which has major effects in the spleen. We will discuss these specific effects in later sections related to inflammation.

The next branch of the vagus after the celiac plexus travels to the small intestine. Once food has been broken down by the chemical and physical churning in the stomach, it enters the small intestine. Here it undergoes further digestive processing by pancreatic digestive enzymes and bile. The function of the small intestine is to break down and absorb most of our macronutrients. These include fats, carbohydrates, and proteins (which are ideally broken down into their component amino acids). The bloodstream receives the macronutrients that have been accepted by the lining cells of the small intestine.

The bite of food that we take (which is called chyme at this point in the digestive process) must be pushed along the winding and coursing length of the small intestine. For this to happen, the vagus nerve activates the smooth muscle cells of the digestive tract by signaling the extensive network of nerves that line the gut, called the enteric nervous system.

Contrary to its name, the small intestine is actually very long, approximately 22 feet long, and significantly longer than the next portion of the digestive tract, the large intestine.

We have an immensely important relationship with the other cells that are living within our digestive tracts. I am speaking of the symbiotic relationship between our human cells and the bacteria that are living in our gut: our microbiome. The vast majority of our bacterial allies live in our large intestine—the thicker, shorter area of the digestive tract. Although these bacteria produce many important vitamins, minerals, and biochemical precursors for us, they can also produce many toxins and gas. We require a system that can keep these bacteria in check and relay signals to our brain regarding the status of digestive tract and microbiome function. So, while the vagus nerve activates smooth muscle cells to push food along the remainder of the digestive tract, it is also the major relay path for the microbiome to speak with the brain. The vagus nerve innervates approximately the first half of the large intestine—the ascending and transverse portions.

The final organ innervated by the vagus nerve is actually two organs, with one located on each side of the body—the kidneys. These organs have a few different functions that are crucial to our health. The kidneys filter fluid out of the body in the form of urine, a combination of uric acid and water, which is then sent down to the bladder. One of the major determinants of this control is blood pressure, which will be discussed further in the next chapter. The vagus nerve is a major controller of the function of the kidneys and thus has a major role in the management of blood pressure.

At the end of its course, the vagus nerve does not simply end. Rather, it forms a final plexus with the parasympathetic nerves that course from the lower end of the spinal cord. These parasympathetic fibers innervate the second half of the large intestine, called the descending and sigmoid colon, as well as the bladder and sex organs.

CHAPTER 3

THE FUNCTIONS OF THE VAGUS NERVE

An optimally functioning VN is absolutely paramount in optimizing health and halting the progression of disease. There are many reasons why, and we will go through some of them in this chapter.

An optimally functioning body is like a symphony orchestra. In a symphony, each of the different instruments have specific parts to play, and optimal harmony can only be reached if each instrument is directed to do its job. The conductor of the orchestra manages to ensure that no instrument is off tune or tempo, as a single mistake could lead to a terrible performance. A conductor that is not holding up their end will lead to a dysfunctional performance as well.

The vagus nerve is the conductor of the human body symphony orchestra. It regulates the function of so many different organs and cells in our body, but it can only do so if it is functioning optimally. It must be able to sense and signal correctly to the many organs and cells of the body. Dysfunctional signaling will lead to a lack of harmony in the body, and eventually to a state of dysfunction and disease.

Let's break down all of the different functions performed by the conductor of the human body orchestra—the vagus nerve.

Sensing Skin of the Ear

As discussed in the previous chapter, the first branch of the vagus nerve is the auricular branch, which is specifically involved in sensing the skin of the auricle, tragus, and external auditory canal of the ear.

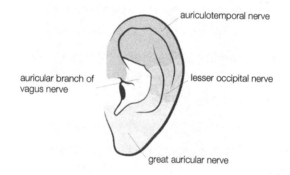

auriculotemporal nerve

auricular branch of
vagus nerve

lesser occipital nerve

great auricular nerve

The function of this branch is purely in sensation, allowing us to feel pressure, touch, temperature, and moisture on the central section of each ear. Clinically this is relevant and quite important, as this is one of the major areas through which the VN can be stimulated using techniques such as acupuncture.

Allowing Food to Be Swallowed

When you are eating a meal, the last thing you are thinking about is the process of swallowing each bite and pausing the breathing reflex so that you don't choke. This important task is managed by the vagus nerve.

The second branch of the VN (the pharyngeal branch) controls the activation of five muscles of the pharynx: the three constrictor muscles at the back of the throat and two other muscles connecting the throat and the soft palate (the soft tissue at the back part of the roof of the mouth). These muscles are involved in the pharyngeal phase of swallowing, which involves pushing chewed food toward the larynx and the esophagus while keeping it out of the trachea, thus keeping the airway clear of food. This branch of the VN also manages the active motor component of the gag reflex.

Clinically this is important, as poor vagus nerve function will lead to coughing and a change in the function of the gag reflex. We can use this reflex to help tone the VN with active exercises and engaging the gag reflex.

Managing Your Airway and Vocal Chords

With every breath you take, are you conscious of the effort required to keep your upper airway open? The muscles involved in this process are also involved in production of your voice. If you've ever wondered what nerve is responsible for ensuring that verbal communication is possible with those around you, it's the vagus!

The third and fourth branches of the VN are the superior and recurrent laryngeal nerves. The superior laryngeal branch is responsible for the muscles above the vocal cords while the recurrent laryngeal branch is responsible for the muscles below the cords.

The superior laryngeal branch carries motor information to some muscles of the larynx and controls vocal pitch. Suboptimal function of the superior laryngeal branch results in a change in pitch. A chronically hoarse voice or an easily fatigued, monotonous voice is a sign of poor vagal tone (signaling capacity) in this branch of the nerve. Irritation of this nerve can also result in severe cough and risk of aspiration (i.e., food or drink entering the trachea through the impaired function of the vocal cords).

The recurrent laryngeal branch carries motor information to the muscles below the vocal cords, allowing sounds to form by opening, closing, and tensioning the vocal cord structures. It also has a sensory component that relays information from the esophagus, trachea, and internal mucous membranes of these structures. Dysfunction of these nerves leads to hoarseness, loss of voice, and trouble breathing during physical activity.

These laryngeal muscles manage the opening, closing, and function of the airway. Any difficulty with breathing or speaking can thus be attributed to decreased vagus nerve function and tone. Breathing and muscle tone of the airway are supremely important for vagal function. Any chronic obstructions to a clear and well-functioning airway will impair the function of and signaling feedback from these muscles, which will negatively affect the function of your vagus nerve.

Controlling Breathing

What about breathing? Well, the vagus has a role in controlling this important task as well. The pulmonary branch of the VN courses to the pulmonary plexus, connects with the sympathetic nervous system, and innervates the trachea and the bronchi of both lungs. The vagus component is a sensory nerve that relays information to the brain regarding lung expansion levels, as well as oxygen and carbon dioxide levels.

In the lungs, the vagus nerve activation slows the breathing rate and deepens the breath. During the rest-and-digest phase, breathing tends to be deeper and come from the diaphragm rather than the accessory muscles for breathing, and the rate of the breath tends to be lower. When a person is transitioning from a fight-or-flight state into a rest-and-digest phase, a slow, deep breath rate will activate the vagus nerve and stimulate the relaxation reflex.

Vagus tone is necessary for opening the airway in the pharynx, larynx, and trachea. The muscles of the pharynx and larynx are innervated by the motor components of VN. Suboptimal activity of these neurons can lead to airway obstruction, as occurs in chronic obstructive pulmonary disease (COPD) and obstructive sleep apnea. Both of these conditions are a sign of low vagal tone and a need for vagus nerve activation. I will even go so far as to say that obstruction of the airways can be a potential root cause of vagus nerve dysfunction—something that will be discussed in much greater detail in later chapters.

Controlling Heart Rate

Your heart beats to get nutrient- and oxygen-filled blood to each of your cells, and to transport toxins to the organs that are able to dispose of them. The VN has a major role in ensuring that the heart rate stays within a comfortable range when the body is not under stress. Without the VN, our heart would not function near its optimal rate.

The vagus nerve is directly connected to the sinoatrial node, which sends electrical signals to the two atria (the thinner chambers at the top of the heart). It is also directly connected to the atrioventricular node, which manages the pumping rate and contraction pressure of the ventricles (the two thicker, lower chambers of the heart).

During times of fight-or-flight, the sympathetic nervous system activates the heart to increase pumping rate and the pressure of the contractions in the two ventricles. When the stressor has passed, rest-and-digest phase takes over and the body moves toward a vagal activation phase. At this time, the parasympathetic fibers of the VN slow the heart rate and actively decrease the pressure of pumping contractions. These fibers work to decrease activity in the heart, allowing the heart to rest and recover from times of stress and severe activation.

Maintaining Optimal Blood Pressure

Blood pressure is a determinant of the amount of fluid present in the bloodstream. The kidneys function to filter fluid and toxins out of the body and are thus the body's major blood pressure manager. The vagus nerve relays information to and from the kidneys to help it manage the flow of water and fluid from within the kidney glomeruli, the basic filtration unit of the kidney, thus managing the overall blood pressure of the body.

When the body is under stress, signals from the blood vessels (specifically the carotid body) are relayed up the brainstem and back down to the kidneys via the vagus and sympathetic nerves. The kidneys then constrict their blood vessels and increase blood pressure by reducing the amount of water being filtered out of the bloodstream. When the body is relaxed, signals from the carotid body tell the kidneys to filter out more water and to dilate the blood vessels to decrease blood pressure.

Hormones are also intimately connected to this process, working with the vagus and sympathetic nerves. However, the immediate control comes from the nerves and the slow, gradual management is determined by the hormones.

High blood pressure is a very common diagnosis and medications are often prescribed to control these levels. High blood pressure can be a sign of overactivation of stress hormones of the adrenal glands, and the stress response, which is mediated through the sympathetic nerves. It is also a very common sign of vagus nerve dysfunction and poor vagal tone.

Controlling the Many Functions of the Liver

The vagus nerve relays much important information to and from the liver, managing its nearly 500 tasks. I will cover just a few of the more commonly known functions in this section.

The liver regulates where blood flows in the body. During times of stress, when the body shifts into fight-or-flight mode, blood flow is pushed toward the arms and legs to increase muscle activation and allow us to fight off an attack, or to run away from it. Blood flow in the liver will decrease, as digestion and blood filtration during this stressful event are not a priority for survival. When the body is relaxed and in the rest-and-digest phase, vagus nerve activation increases and blood flow to the liver will increase. During these times, digestion, filtration of blood, and other functions for cellular thriving are prioritized.

The vagus nerve also controls the cells in the liver that are responsible for producing bile and bile salts, as well as transporting bile into the gallbladder and small intestine. It has been shown that when the vagus nerve is active, these cells, called cholangiocytes, are active and increase the flow of bile into the gallbladder for storage.

Bile performs multiple functions for the liver and the body. The liver detoxifies fat-soluble toxins through a two-step process, creating a water-soluble waste product that must be released. Bile holds these toxins that have been rendered harmless and are ready to be released from the body through the digestive tract via our stool. Stool is only one of three routes by which the waste products are released. The other methods of waste elimination are as urine via the kidneys or as sweat via the skin.

Bile salts, the effective component of bile, have another role. When bile is released into the small intestine, it releases waste product and bile salts. The bile salts are required to escort triglycerides (molecules of fat) from the digestive tract, across the enterocytes (the cells that line the small intestine), and into the bloodstream. Without being escorted by bile salts, fats are not able to be absorbed, which is a bad thing, because fats and cholesterol have numerous vital functions in the body. This results in fatty stools, as well. The role of the vagus nerve in this function is to activate cholangiocytes and to open the flow of bile from the liver into the gallbladder, as well as from the gallbladder into the small intestine, ensuring that fat can be absorbed by the enterocytes.

Activating Gall Bladder Emptying

Once the liver has produced bile and the cholangiocytes have sent that bile into the gallbladder, it is stored and matures, like a fine wine, until it is needed. Upon eating a meal, the taste buds in the tongue and rest of the mouth send signals to the brain, letting our body know about the macronutrients that it senses as part of each bite and the entirety of the snack or meal. If the central nervous system indicates that fats are being consumed, then the vagus nerve signals the liver and gallbladder that bile will be needed soon.

Upon receiving this signal, the gallbladder will activate the smooth muscle cells in its lining and pump the bile out through the bile duct into the small intestine to aid in fat digestion. Without this vagus nerve signal, the gallbladder will remain full and not pump out the necessary bile—a condition known as obstructive cholestasis.

One of the most common procedures taking place in hospitals and clinics in North America is the removal of the gallbladder, called cholecystectomy. Surgery to remove a gallbladder due to obstruction, such as gallstones, is often the first option provided to patients that begin to experience the pain associated with obstructive cholestasis. Unfortunately, most patients are not given the opportunity to determine the root cause of this condition.

Gallstones are a painful problem that can affect the gallbladder. Gallstones form in the gallbladder following a long period of low vagus nerve function, which would prevent the gallbladder from adequately pumping out bile and bile salts. When bile salts remain in the gallbladder for a long time, they begin to crystallize and form stones. This tends to happen with a lack of vagus nerve activation and is an early sign of dysfunction in this nerve. It has been shown in clinical settings that in early cases of this condition, gallstones can be released when the vagus nerve begins to function at a higher level. Performing some of the vagus nerve activation exercises and therapies that we will discuss in later chapters can be very useful for those dealing with gallbladder pain due to cholestasis and gallstone formation.

Managing Hunger and Satiety

Satiety is reached when our brain receives signals from the vagus nerve. In order to be satiated, we require signals from the liver, indicating that we have enough fat, protein, and carbohydrates in the body. The metabolism of carbohydrates and fats both occur in the liver.

In terms of carbohydrate metabolism, the following control is mediated by the vagus nerve: When blood sugar levels gradually decrease, afferent vagal fibers in the liver increase activity and signal to the brain that the liver cells require more carbohydrates. This pathway does not signal sudden changes in blood sugar, though; these are directly sensed in the brain.

A hormone called glucagon-like peptide 1 (GLP-1) is released by the small intestine as a response to increased blood sugar levels, which the body translates as satiety. Decreasing GLP-1 levels signal the vagus nerve, which in turn manages a slow reduction in blood sugar. Many pharmaceutical companies are now producing medications that work on the GLP-1 pathway to help manage hunger; however, this can be managed in your own body by activating the vagus nerve.

The vagus nerve offers another path to feelings of satiety. After eating a meal, vagal afferent neurons send information to the brain regarding the amount of fats that have made their way to the liver, especially triglycerides and linoleic acid. This activates vagus nerve function, sending a signal to the brain that produces a feeling of satiety and a desire to stop eating.

An underactive vagus nerve may not be able to effectively send this signal, leading to continuous feelings of hunger, lack of satiety, and overeating during meal time. When the VN is working effectively, it will take less than 15 to 20 minutes to feel full after a meal. If you know someone who is lacking the feeling of satiety and their hunger persists even after a large meal, they are likely suffering from VN dysfunction.

Managing Blood Sugar and Insulin Levels

Insulin resistance and type II diabetes levels are growing at exorbitant rates. Obesity and the aptly named diabesity—concurrent diabetes and obesity—are major symptoms of an unhealthy lifestyle. Weight issues and blood sugar control problems are major signs that something in your body is working suboptimally.

During times of stress, our bodies shift their balance toward the sympathetic nervous system and release more of the adrenal stress hormones, specifically cortisol. The primary effect of cortisol is to increase blood sugar by stimulating a process called gluconeogenesis, which is when new glucose is created from fat and protein stored in the liver.

In short bursts, using the sympathetic nervous system is important for keeping us alive and allowing us to survive. This fight-or-flight system evolved in response to external threats to our survival—think of our ancestors needing to run away from a saber-toothed tiger. In this situation, when the stressor is approaching us, our bodies must shift into survival mode. We must either fight the threat, or take flight and run as fast as possible.

To facilitate the fight-or-flight response, our skeletal muscles require significant energy-forming resources—preferably, the fastest-acting and most easily accessible way to form cellular energy, which would allow us to survive the threat. For short-term fuel, our bodies can quickly produce glucose, using gluconeogenesis, and send it through the bloodstream. The sympathetic nervous system quickly shifts blood flow toward the muscles of the arms and legs to make us extra strong and fast, while shifting it away from the digestive tract and kidneys. We are then able to use our muscles effectively to fight the threat or to run away as fast as humanly possible.

The problem with this system is that it is often active for longer periods than is absolutely necessary. Under the chronic stress we experience at work and home, with our finances,

Activate your VAGUS NERVE

relationships, friends, and families, and due to biochemical stressors and stealth infections, our bodies tend to stay in the fight-or-flight state for significantly longer than it should, and we do not shift back to the rest-and-digest state in which the parasympathetic recovery system is primarily active. The inability to shift back leads the liver to continuously produce glucose, leading to higher blood sugar levels in the longer term. In response to high blood sugar levels, the pancreas is activated to form insulin. Insulin is the messenger that signals each of our cells to take in glucose from the blood and use it to form energy.

How We Process Insulin

I like to think of insulin like Girl Scouts who will come by, knock on your door, and offer you cookies once in a while. If each house on your block is a muscle cell, then each time the blood sugar levels increase, insulin will come knocking. In an ideal scenario, the Girl Scouts will knock on your door once or twice per day, and not very loudly. In this scenario, your door plays the role of the insulin receptors on the muscle cell. Each time they knock on your door, you answer it and gladly accept the treat that is being offered. Initially you would be sensitive to the knock at the door, just as our cells are ideally sensitive to insulin.

When blood sugar levels surge and spike up very high, the Girl Scouts come and pound on your door with all of their might, as they need you to take the cookies as soon as possible so they can move on to the next house and do the same thing. This occurs when the scouts have a wagon full of cookies and need to sell them all as quickly as possible before their next shipment arrives. I imagine they would be pushy and ask you to

The Functions of the Vagus Nerve

take multiple boxes, rather than your regular order. Once in a while, this would be okay and you would not feel pressured or upset by this. It would become an issue, however, if they came pounding on your door three, four, and even five times per day. If this pounding on the door persisted multiple times per day, each day for a week, you would likely become annoyed. Eventually, you would even stop answering the door. You would have become resistant to the Girl Scouts in the same way that our cells become resistant to insulin.

When our cells become resistant to insulin, they simply stop answering the door for insulin. They will no longer take in the treats that insulin is offering. This leads to higher insulin levels and higher blood sugar levels.

If this same issue starts to occur with each house on your street, and then with each house in your neighborhood, then the Girl Scouts will eventually have no choice but to stop coming to the neighborhood. As their sales levels decrease, the cookie suppliers will stop sending them cookies and will send them to a storage facility instead. The storage facility is code for our fat storage cells, called adipocytes or adipose tissue. This tissue is located throughout the body, but the body has most effectively placed the majority of it in the central area of the body: the belly. This allows the arms and legs to function under times of fight-or-flight, when muscle strength is still required.

In this analogy, if the Girl Scouts stop coming to your neighborhood and knocking at your door, the supply of insulin has essentially burnt out and is no longer effective. This is type II diabetes, which occurs when the pancreas has burnt out after producing so much insulin for such a long time. It could no longer handle all the surges in blood sugar and thus stops working. Diabetic patients are often prescribed medications that either stimulate insulin sensitivity or are given insulin itself to help manage their blood sugar. Chronic stress, chronic overeating, and a high-sugar diet are often at the root of this issue and are some of the most common reasons for the development of obesity, insulin resistance, and diabetes.

So what does all of this have to do with the vagus nerve? Just as we discussed earlier, our bodies are under long-term and chronic stress, which leads to vagus nerve inactivity and dysfunction. Under optimal circumstances, our bodies should spend the vast majority of their time in the rest, digest, and recovery system that is signaled by the vagus nerve. When this system is active, it should help to increase insulin sensitivity and allow the liver to decrease gluconeogenesis. The function of the liver will shift toward digestion and filtration of toxins from the bloodstream. The VN will also send signals to the liver asking it to form a signaling molecule called hepatic insulin sensitizing substance, which increases insulin sensitivity and glucose storage in the muscle cells.

The important thing to remember is that lower blood sugar levels are needed to activate the rest-and-digest system and increase our insulin sensitivity. The vagus nerve, when activated, is also highly involved in managing blood sugar levels through the pancreas, which is a major trigger for the production and secretion of insulin.

The islet cells of the pancreas produce and secrete insulin in response to increasing levels of blood glucose. As glucose increases, insulin secretion increases. A spike in blood sugar levels will lead directly to a spike in the release of insulin, and chronic repetitive spikes will lead to insulin resistance and eventually diabetes, as described earlier. A hormone called cholecystokinin (CCK), which is released in the gut following a meal, directly triggers the vagus nerve, which later signals the islet cells to release insulin as necessary.

Vagus function must be optimized to ensure proper signaling from the gut to the brain and from the brain to the pancreas. Less than optimal function will over time lead to a disease state due to chronic dysfunctional signaling. We must be able to activate the parasympathetic vagus system with regularity to prevent insulin resistance and eventually blood sugar dys-regulation and diabetes.

Managing the Release of Digestive Enzymes from the Pancreas

The pancreas is not just involved in blood sugar control; it is also highly responsible for producing and secreting digestive enzymes into the small intestine in response to a meal.

When we eat, our taste buds and sensory cells in the small intestine send signals to the brain that determine the specific macronutrients that are present in the meal. Does the meal contain protein, fat, and/or carbohydrate? How much of each has entered the digestive tract, and how quickly? Once the answers to these questions are determined, the vagus signals the pancreas to release specific digestive enzymes—proteases, lipases, and amylases—to aid in the breakdown of these macro-nutrients, allowing for digestion and eventually the proper use of these nutrients by our cells.

In response to higher levels of protein, the pancreas secretes proteases to help break down the bonds between the amino acids that make up the proteins. In response to higher levels

Activate your VAGUS NERVE

of fats, the pancreas secretes lipases to help break down triglycerides into cholesterol and free fatty acids. Lastly, in response to higher carbohydrate levels, amylase is secreted to help break down complex carbohydrates into simple sugars.

Without this process, our bodies would not be able to absorb the important macronutrients required for cellular function. Amino acids are mostly involved in creating new proteins within our cells, including protein and peptide hormones, neurotransmitters, receptors, and certain intracellular signaling molecules. The free fatty acids and simple sugars are used primarily for energy production, while the cholesterol component of the fats is used as the precursor to steroid hormones such as estrogen, testosterone, and cortisol. All of these molecules are necessary for cellular function, so an optimally functioning pancreas is required to ensure that these molecules make it into the body.

Managing Gut Motor Function

Getting food from the mouth to the opposite end of the digestive tract is an important role of the vagus. Upon taking a bite of food, we chew that food down in our mouth until it is physically capable of being swallowed and transported through the remainder of the digestive tract.

As soon as that food, or bolus, hits the back of the mouth—the pharynx—it is the job of the vagus nerve to push it to the next area. For this to happen, the sensors and muscles lining the digestive tract must be functioning correctly. As each bite reaches the back of the throat, it elicits a stretch reflex in the smooth muscles that signals the brainstem through the vagus nerve, letting it know where the bolus is located. In response, the VN signals the smooth muscle cells to engage in motor activity and push the bolus of food along in a downward direction. This process is known as peristalsis.

This seemingly simple function is actually very complex and necessary, as the digestive tract is quite long. Movement along the digestive tract is required for us to extract nutrition from our food and push out any unwanted visitors.

A poorly toned VN can be a root cause for impaired movement of a bolus through the tract. Chronic constipation and diarrhea are certainly signs of poor vagal tone and a lack of necessary activation of these muscles and nerve. Some of the biggest issues causing this problem are that we don't chew our food well enough and that we eat in a rush and much too quickly. I call this the drive-through effect, as we are eating in a rush while in a stress-filled environment. We are trying to activate a rest-and-digest process while in a fight-or-flight state.

For now, it is necessary to understand that food cannot move along this path—from the pharynx, to the esophagus, through the stomach, into all three parts of the small intestine, and against gravity in the ascending and transverse colon—without a correctly functioning vagus nerve.

Managing the Activity of the Immune System

Consider this question: Would you drive a car that did not have working brakes? A car has the important function of safely getting you from point A to point B, and your immune system has the important function of keeping you safe from invading cells and proteins. And just as a car needs a system of checks and balances such as brakes, the immune cells in your body need a similar set of checks and balances.

Without its brakes, the immune system can run amok and begin attacking human cells, which can lead to autoimmunity, or it can even stop attacking tumor cells, leading to cancer. Without brakes, a car can be a very dangerous tool. Without a system to keep it in check, the immune system can also be quite dangerous. Enter, the vagus nerve.

Overview of the Immune System

The immune system is the defensive system of the body. It protects you from invaders and unwanted toxins that can, and often do, lead to unfavorable health conditions. This system includes white blood cells that send out sensors to check for the presence of invaders in the body. In an optimally functioning scenario, they roam through the bloodstream detecting proteins and organisms that have entered the body and send signals to other immune cells whose function it is to eliminate these invaders that should not be present.

There are multiple different types of white blood cells, also known as leukocytes, in the immune system, including monocytes, macrophages, neutrophils, mast cells, and dendritic cells, collectively known as phagocytes; as well as basophils, eosinophils, lymphocytes (T cells and B cells), and natural killer cells.

"Phagocytes" literally means "cells that eat." When they identify dead or dying human cells, unwanted bacteria, and dangerous proteins that should not be present, they activate and begin to literally engulf the unwanted cells or proteins, beginning a process called phagocytosis. They break these

The Functions of the Vagus Nerve

invaders down and create debris that is later filtered out of the blood in the immune organs and liver. Each phagocyte senses different invaders and has a different way of breaking them down, but these cells are all essential for an effectively balanced and functioning immune system.

In addition to phagocytosis, mast cells are also highly involved in allergy and anaphylaxis, as they contain and release granules rich in histamine. These are likely to be hyperactive in a person dealing with chronic allergies and similar reactions. Mast cells are shown to be highly active in autoimmunity by ensuring that we experience the symptoms of the condition. They are also one of the only immune cells located in both the gut and the brain. When mast cells are overactivated in the brain, the nerves of the brain can become more sensitive to pain, leading to brain inflammation. Similarly, when these cells are activated in the gut, they make the nerves of the gut more sensitive to pain and lead to gut inflammation around the nerves, which will impair the normal movement of gut motility (peristalsis). As we will discuss soon, the vagus nerve is the major controller of gut motility, and thus, mast cell hyperactivation can be a trigger for vagus nerve dysfunction.

Basophils are responsible for inflammatory reactions during an immune response and, like mast cells, are involved in conditions that cause allergic symptoms such as anaphylaxis, asthma, atopic dermatitis, and hay fever. They can be triggered by parasites and allergies, both of which can commonly occur and enter the body through the digestive tract or through broken skin.

Eosinophils are responsible for reacting to and combating parasites and infections. Like basophils, they are also known to be involved in allergies and asthma. Low-grade, chronic infections by parasites or bacteria can lead to overstimulation of eosinophils, which have been shown to trigger asthmatic and allergic symptoms. Most commonly, these infections affect us and enter our body through the digestive tract.

Natural killer cells are the major cells involved in combating viruses and tumor growth in the body. They do not require sensors to identify human cells vs. invader cells, hence the name natural killers. Dysfunction of these cells may lead to tumor growth and a decreased ability for the body to identify and combat these cancerous growths.

To do their job, the vast majority of leukocytes produce sensors that roam the internal environment of the body. These sensors are called antibodies, or immunoglobulins. There are five different types of these sensors—immunoglobulin A (IgA), IgE, IgG, IgM, and IgD. Each of these sensors has a different role and a different speed at which it signals for the white blood cells to react.

IgG is the most abundant sensor and is found on the surface of mature immune cells. Its function is to identify cells and proteins that should not be present, and to activate a pathway that leads to inflammation and immune activation.

IgA is the second most abundant sensor, and a specific subset of IgA (called secretory IgA) is sent out in our bodily fluids such as breast milk, saliva, and secretions of the digestive tract. Secretory IgA is important in identifying potential threats in the digestive tract, including the mouth. High levels of IgA signal the presence of bacteria, viruses, parasites, and yeast, while low levels of IgA signal that the immune system is dysfunctioning due to chronic activation by these same invaders. I measure secretory IgA levels for my patients to determine their current state of immune function and activation. This is a very important and useful tool used in functional medicine practice.

IgM, IgE, and IgD are far less common. They are found on the surface of mature immune cells and have a similar function to IgG.

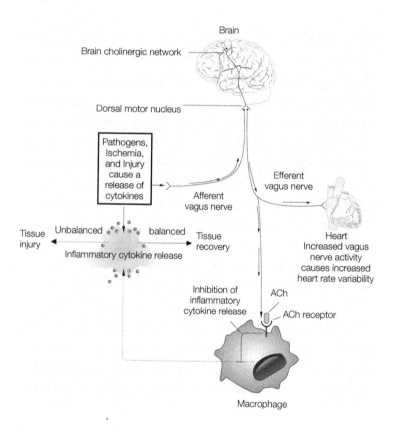

The system to keep immune cells in check is mediated through the vagus nerve. A properly functioning vagus nerve is required to set off an important pathway called the cholinergic anti-inflammatory pathway. When active, the pathway keeps the immune system in check and pumps the brakes

Activate your VAGUS NERVE

when necessary. Vagus innervation to the immune organs, such as the thymus, spleen, and gut, are highly involved in activating the pathway. Before you learn about the pathway itself, it's important to learn about how these important organs work in the immune system.

The thymus is the primary lymphatic organ. It primarily produces T cells, white blood cells that seek and destroy foreign invaders. The vagus nerve sends a branch to the thymus to activate it, while sympathetic fibers that run to this organ can deactivate it. On average, the thymus is fully functional until we hit puberty, at which time it begins to shrink and decrease in both size and function. This process is called "involution of the thymus." Recent research has shown that our high-stress lifestyle and hyperactivation of the sympathetic branches can lead to deactivation of the thymus at an earlier age. This is believed to be a root cause of autoimmune conditions and increased risk of infection by bacteria, viruses, and other invaders.

Earlier in our lives, our immune systems learn and grow to create a system that helps to protect us from infection by bacteria, viruses, and other invaders that should not enter our bodies. This is a dynamic system, one that requires years of training and preparation in dealing with invaders of the body. Overstimulation of the thymus can occur via parasympathetic fibers and lead to excessive growth of the organ; however, this is not very common. The far more common issue is that there is a higher level of sympathetic activation, which actually deactivates the organ prematurely.

As long as you have a strong functioning thymus, your body is protected as it develops. The thymus acts as a school or training facility for immune cells, the police officers of the body. As long as this training facility is active and fully funded, it continues to pump out fully qualified and highly intelligent police officers that protect our cells from invaders. When the funding to this school decreases, fewer, more poorly trained officers are released, and the level of protection withers, putting us at much higher risk of infection by invaders.

This demonstrates why we have a higher risk of infectious disease as we get older and also why we have a higher risk of autoimmune conditions following highly stressful life events. In an autoimmune condition, our immune cells are not as well suited to distinguishing invading cells from our own cells. As we age, we are exposed to stressful life situations, and thus rates of autoimmune conditions increase, including, but certainly not limited to, Hashimoto's thyroiditis, rheumatoid arthritis, multiple sclerosis, Crohn's disease, ulcerative colitis, and many others.

The spleen is the next checkpoint for the cells of the immune system. Think of the spleen as the filter for the white and red blood cells. It ensures that only qualified, fully trained immune cells are present in the bloodstream and other tissues of the body. It will remove and filter out any cells that are nearing the end of their optimal functioning period. The spleen functions as a check and balance for the immune cells of the bloodstream. When functioning optimally, it ensures that the immune system protects against invaders while not overtly acting against our own cells. The vagus nerve relays information back and forth between the central nervous system to let our bodies know which cells are being filtered out of the blood.

Activate your VAGUS NERVE

As with the thymus and so many other organs, the parasympathetic activity of the vagus is required to keep the spleen active, while the sympathetic activity will temporarily decrease or shut down splenic activity. Chronic stress or activation of the sympathetic branches will undoubtedly lead to chronically decreased levels of spleen function, and in turn, poor filtration of white and red blood cells. This leads to a higher likelihood of autoimmune disease, as the roaming less-qualified "police officers" are not kept in check and are unable to distinguish between invaders and our own cellular proteins.

When a damaging event occurs in the body, or when invaders are detected, the immune cells closest to the area assess the threat and release proteins called cytokines to attract additional cells that will aid in the immune response. These cytokines are detected by vagus nerve afferent fibers that send signals back to the brain to inform it about the type of inflammation that is building up. Recent research has even shown that the vagus nerve can differentiate between cytokines.

The gut is the most common area through which invaders can enter the body, and as such, the vast majority of our immune cells are located in the lining of the gut. They are held in small pockets throughout the digestive tract, which we affectionately refer to as gut-associated lymphoid tissue (GALT). In the gut, the functions of the vagus nerve are quite extensive and necessary to ensure optimal health. It helps regulate immune and inflammatory responses, allow us to create memories, and relay information between the gut bacteria and the brain. These roles are discussed in the next three sections.

Managing Inflammation in the Gut

Continuing the discussion of the effect of the vagus nerve on immune responses in the gut, we will discuss what is likely the most important role of the vagus—the cholinergic anti-inflammatory pathway. Through this pathway, the vagus nerve sends signals to the cells of the immune system throughout the body, but particularly strong signals in the gut, using the neurotransmitter acetylcholine (ACh). These signals are meant to calm immune activation and decrease inflammation.

Afferent vagus activity in the thymus and the spleen has been shown to increase in response to stressors including lipopolysaccharide (LPS), a toxin produced and released by one of two types of bacteria, and invaders such as bacteria, viruses, and parasites in our gut. At the same time, the sympathetic branch of the nervous system, the fight-or-flight response, ensures that immune cells are ready to target the invaders. When immune cells first detect the presence of these unwanted stressors in the gut, they send a signal to the GALT, which activates a stress response and the sympathetic nerves. The sympathetic nerves then signal the neurotransmitter norepinephrine (NE), also referred to as adrenaline. NE activates the immune cells, which become highly reactive to invaders and stressors. This system is highly important, but as with all important systems, brakes are necessary for optimal function.

Parasympathetic activity in the vast majority of the gut is run through the vagus nerve. Its role is to keep inflammation and immune response in check. The vagus nerve and its branches send out ACh in the gut and other areas of the body to counteract the pro-inflammatory response of the sympathetic nerves and norepinephrine. When working optimally, there is a

Activate your VAGUS NERVE

perfect balance between sympathetic NE secretion and parasympathetic ACh secretion. This keeps our health in check by stimulating an immune response when necessary and turning it off when unnecessary. Control of a function comes from the ability to shut it off.

ACh is released from the vagus nerve in response to higher levels of stress and immune activity. The release is amplified significantly and effectively by the enteric nervous system, a collection of nerve cells in the gut that is so vast, it is also known as the second brain. Some argue that the enteric nervous system is more important than the brain in our head because much of our health is dictated by the interaction between this system and our microbiome.

An important receptor found on the surface of most white blood cells—the alpha-7 nicotinic acetylcholine receptor—facilitates the effect of ACh on immune cells. This receptor works to decrease activation and slow the immune response when it is not required. It is crucial in balancing the parasympathetic and sympathetic activation of the inflammatory response in the gut.

Relaying Information from the Microbiome

Research into the microbiome has become the greatest revelation into our health in centuries. We are learning new amazing things each day regarding the population of bacteria in our gut and its impact on our health and biochemistry. This population is responsible for the vast majority of our nutrient health, neurotransmitters, our mood, and even how our brains work.

There are nearly 100 trillion bacterial cells in our digestive tract, way more than the number of human cells in our body. These bacteria have a specific population breakdown that can affect nearly every aspect of our health and well-being. Signal relaying from the gut bacteria to the brain takes place most quickly through the vagus nerve and is supplemented by the bloodstream and hormonal systems.

Of all the other organs and systems controlled through the vagus, we are most likely to feel the gut and bacterial changes. We can "tune in" to our gut and what is happening in there, unlike with our heart, liver, or spleen. The most common example of this is a craving. As stated in a great book called *The Psychobiotic Revolution*, written by Scott Anderson, John Cryan, and Ted Dinan, "Your cravings are often just committee memos sent up from your gut microbes. They contain a complete list of the carbs, sugars, and fats they are looking for."

The book continues to discuss the example of Bifidobacterium (a.k.a. Bifido), a genus of bacteria that is found in high proportion in our gut: "Some microbes, especially our friendly Bifido species, produce butyrate, which feeds and heals the lining of your gut. Butyrate can make its way to the brain, where it can induce a good mood, dampen inflammation, or encourage the production of a brain-growth hormone. All these changes can improve your mood and even help you think better."

Another type of bacteria that is discussed in this book are in the Lactobacillus (a.k.a. Lacto) genus. Anderson, Cryan, and Dinan elaborate: "In studies with people suffering from IBS, it was found that some Lacto species actually manipulate the opioid and cannabinoid receptors in the brain, acting almost like a shot of morphine. Like the addiction to a runner's high, this kind of reaction can lead to cravings for whatever food your Lacto microbes prefer. You might think your cravings are all in your mind, but chances are they begin with the bacteria in your gut."

Once we realize that cravings and signals regarding the foods our bacteria want are actually being relayed by the vagus nerve and through our bloodstream, it is possible to take back control of our choices and make dietary changes that can have a beneficial effect on our microbiome and our overall health.

Allowing Us to Create Memories

Recent research has shown that the presence of gut bacteria is necessary for development and maturation of the enteric nervous system as well as the central nervous system. As discussed earlier, the vagus nerve is highly involved in the relay of microbiome information from the gut bacteria to the brain. This chain of communication may be responsible for activating production of a protein called brain-derived neurotrophic factor (BDNF). Activation of BDNF leads to increased neuronal connectivity, and most importantly, the production of memories in the brain.

This means that without gut bacteria and a healthy functioning vagus nerve, it may be difficult to form new memories and create new neuronal connections. To an even greater extent, this means that if you have an optimally functioning vagus nerve, you will likely be able to form greater memories and associations with the world around you and those who are important to you.

During our fetal development, we produce barriers to protect us from external threats. The gut-blood barrier is one such barrier, protecting us from bacteria (both good and bad) that may want to invade. It is formed from the same cells that produce our blood-brain barrier. This means that any inflammation that occurs in the gut and causes the gut barrier to break down also has the ability to break down the blood-brain barrier.

Have you ever walked into a room and forgotten why you went into that particular room? Have you ever tried to say something very simple but couldn't find the right words to say? These issues are commonly called "brain fog" and are caused by higher-than-optimal levels of inflammation in the brain. Brain fog occurs when the blood-brain barrier has broken down slightly and inflammatory signals are allowed to enter the brain tissue, decreasing the function of neurons.

Brain fog indicates the presence of inflammation in the brain, caused by a less-than-optimal functioning blood-brain barrier, and thus, poor functioning gut lining, or leaky gut.

***

Vagus function is clearly much more important than simple biochemistry and physiology. How does it manage to do it all at once?

CHAPTER 4

HOW THE VAGUS NERVE MANAGES IT ALL

Neurons function to send signals to other cells within the body. These signals may be for muscle function, proprioception (reception of stimuli), active thought in the brain, and of course, automatic functions that take place via the autonomic nervous system. For a neuron's signal to affect the intended cells, three things need to occur:

1. The neuron needs to send an electrically charged signal throughout its entire length.

2. The neuron needs to release a protein called a neurotransmitter into the space between itself and the cell it wants to affect.

3. The neurotransmitter must fit into a protein receptor on the surface of, and elicit activity within, the next cell.

In the case of the vagus nerve, many neuron signals need to work optimally so it can manage all of its tasks.

Sending the Signal Through Neurons

As you read in Chapter 1, approximately 80 percent of the signals being sent along the vagus are from the organs to the brain—afferent signals. You learned that these signals relay information about the current state of function, whether anything is going wrong, and what needs immediate attention. The vagus, which is the longest nerve in the body, communications information from the liver about detoxification, bile production, and blood sugar balance; from the digestive tract about the digestive process, movement of food, and the microbiome; and most importantly, from the immune system cells and organs about their state of function. It also relays information from the heart and lungs regarding their activity levels and any impairments that are taking place.

The signals are sent through very long axons and dendrites, the long arms and legs of neuron cells. It is very important that the signals are able to relay strongly from one end of the neuron to the other. As I'm sure you can understand, these signals have to travel distances as far as the intestines and kidneys to the brain. To send these signals effectively, the vagus neurons need a level of insulation. When an electrical cord carries a signal through a metal wire, that cord needs insulation in the form of a material wrapped around it that does not conduct electricity, such as plastic or rubber. This ensures that the electrical charge remains inside the cord. And, if a wire is frayed, the signal will not be sent strongly and may dissipate and weaken before it gets to the brain.

Our cells store fat to insulate nerves to ensure that signals move quickly and effectively from one end to the other. Most of the nerves in our body are protected by Schwann cells, and the vagus nerve is no exception. Schwann cells create an insulating barrier around neurons called a myelin sheath that protects signals and ensures nerves function effectively. Any damage to these Schwann cells can actually lead to "fraying" of the insulation and ineffective signaling along the nerve. We begin to develop this myelin sheath while we are still in our mother's womb, at 24 weeks of development. The myelin continues to develop until approximately 40 weeks, when we are at full term. This rate of myelination remains approximately the same until we reach adolescent age, when it begins to decline. The Schwann cells and myelin sheath ensure that signals make it from one end of the vagus to the other.

Releasing the Chemical Messenger

Once an electrical signal reaches the end of a neuron at the area called the terminal axon, the signal creates a charge that induces a neurotransmitter to be released from the cell. There are many different neurotransmitters in the body, some of which I have mentioned previously, including NE and ACh. The vagus nerve almost exclusively uses ACh as its neurotransmitter.

ACh needs to be built from two separate structures: acetyl coenzyme A (acetyl-CoA) and choline. Through different metabolic processes, glucose and free fatty acids are broken down into acetyl-CoA. These metabolic reactions require specific micronutrients to function optimally. To metabolize free fatty acids, our cells require sufficient amounts of carnitine and vitamin B2, while to metabolize glucose, our cells require high quantities of vitamin B1, vitamin B3, chromium, lipoic acid, and coenzyme Q10. Unfortunately, as testing performed in my office shows, our bodies are commonly lacking these nutrients. Urinary organic acid functional lab testing can help ensure that this process is occurring smoothly and nutrients are present to fulfill these obligations.

Choline, on the other hand, is an organic compound that comes from certain amino acids. It is considered an essential nutrient for humans, meaning it cannot be produced within our body—it must be taken in as part of the diet. The foods that contain this compound in the highest quantities are egg yolks, soy, and beef, chicken, and turkey livers. It is often a component of soy lecithin, which is found in many food products as an additive.

Acetyl-CoA and choline come together to form acetylcholine in the neurons. ACh is released from the vagus neuron axons so it can affect the various cells and organs that are controlled by this nerve. This process ensures that the second requirement of nerve function is fulfilled—release of a neurotransmitter into the space near the desired cell to be effected. For this reason, having effective sources of acetyl-CoA and choline are very important to our health.

Receiving the Signal in the Next Cell

When a nerve releases a neurotransmitter, it does not immediately have an effect on the next cell. There is actually a very small space or gap between the end of the neuron axon and the cell that is receiving the signals, called a synapse. The neurotransmitter is released into the synapse and must be present in high enough quantities to find its way to receptor proteins on the next cell.

In the case of the vagus nerve, ACh is released into the synapse and binds to receptor proteins on the surface of many different types of cells. The receptor protein that these cells use to receive ACh signals from vagus are either the fast-acting nicotinic acetylcholine receptors (nAChR) or the slower muscarinic acetylcholine receptors (mAChR). Each receptor cell must have its own specific type of AChR to receive the signals from the vagus and induce a response within the individual cell type. Most organs and non-neuron cells express the nicotinic receptor, while other neurons in the central nervous system tend to express the muscarinic versions.

Certain circumstances can cause receptor production to be decreased or even increased on receptor cells. One of the most important is the presence of LPS, which gets sent in by opportunistic gut bacteria and causes the breakdown of cells of the intestine. In the presence of LPS, the gene that holds the blueprint for this protein has the potential to become significantly more or significantly less active. This can explain why some people are highly sensitive to inflammatory gut changes and some are less sensitive. Regardless of sensitivity levels, LPS is a trigger for changes to this gene and causes issues for receptor protein concentrations.

PART 2

WHAT COULD GO WRONG IN VAGUS?

Having gone through all of the different and significantly important tasks that the vagus nerve performs, it is easy to see that if VN function is not optimal, your health could suffer.

Imagine, for a moment, the charging wire for your cell phone. If the wire had one of three different problems, your cell phone would not receive adequate power from the outlet that you have plugged it into. These three problems include:

1. the plug not being properly fit into the wall outlet,

2. the wire not successfully attaching to the charging port of your cell phone, and

3. the wire itself being damaged, frayed, or bent.

Any of these three issues would result in slower-than-normal charging of your cell phone and a significant level of frustration.

The vagus nerve has similar points of damage; however, the results of dysfunctional signaling in the nerve have significantly more damaging and far-reaching effects and can result in the need for diagnosis and treatment with conventional medicine. Keep in mind as we go through Part 2 that vagus nerve tone can be improved and fixed in a vast majority of cases. There is hope if you or a loved one is suffering from the effects of dysfunctional information relay.

In the following chapters, we will go over the most common mechanisms that lead to dysfunction of the vagus nerve and discuss the way these dysfunctions might show up as symptoms.

CHAPTER 5

DYSFUNCTIONAL BREATHING

The first and most common cause of dysfunctional signaling in the vagus nerve is dysfunctional breathing.

Immediately upon exiting our mother's womb, we are tasked with taking our first breath of air. While in the womb, our hearts are already breathing and our digestive tracts are already working thanks to the support of our mothers. Breathing is the first task we are given when we are born, and it's the only thing that our tiny, brand-new bodies have to do to survive outside of the warm, comfortable environment in which we grew and developed for approximately 40 weeks.

The doctor or midwife can help us with this initially by clearing our airway, allowing for the free flow of air into the lungs and the contraction and relaxation of our diaphragm muscle. They support this task by clearing fluid that may be obstructing the pathway. This fluid usually enters the airway and lungs when we take some practice breaths very late in our fetal development. The diaphragm must learn to contract and relax, as it is the controlling factor necessary for the act of breathing.

The vagus nerve has no effect on the diaphragm. It is controlled by the phrenic nerve, which originates in the neck (from levels 3–5 of the cervical spine) and courses adjacent to the vagus into the thorax and past the lungs and heart before it reaches the most important muscle for the task of breathing.

Once our airways are cleared, the task of taking that first breath begins. Our diaphragm contracts and creates a vacuum effect in our thorax, forcing our lungs to expand and take in the external air that contains oxygen, among other gases. The vagus nerve signals the expansion of our lungs to the brainstem, and we realize that our mother is no longer providing physical support for the oxygen that we need. That task is now ours for the rest of our lives. Our diaphragm then relaxes and pushes the air out from the lungs and through the trachea, then out through our nose and mouth. The process of breathing has begun.

As a baby, we learn to breathe in the automatic and correct way. The next time you are around a healthy infant or toddler, take a moment and watch how they breathe. What you will notice is that for them to take a breath in, their diaphragm must contract, and in doing so, they will actually expand their belly in the process. Diaphragmatic breathing is the process of using this major muscle rather than accessory muscles for breathing.

Take a moment right now, put one hand on your belly and one hand on your chest, close your eyes, and take a deep breath.

I'm serious... test yourself to see if you are breathing correctly, right now!

Did your belly expand as you took this deep breath or did your shoulders rise to accommodate the expansion of your lungs?

As we grow and develop through childhood and enter our teen years, we observe those around us with the greatest of admiration and the desire for emulation. We want to look like and act like those around us; we tend to copy the mannerisms of people we look up to. Oftentimes, these people are in the media and presented to us in a superficial way. In the North American social media–crazed society, how you look is considered to be one of the most important factors of who you are. It is an unfortunate truth but a serious observation that many others and I have come across. We are taught in childhood and our adolescent lives that thinner is better and that our belly size is a reflection of who we are.

When we begin to take these thoughts into consideration and compare them to how we look and feel as teenagers, we actually alter our breathing patterns. The consistent expansion and contraction of our abdomen is not considered attractive, so we learn to breathe in a different way. We start to use our accessory muscles for breathing—the backup muscles that are more important and useful during stressful situations. We begin to control the expansion of the thorax and creation of the vacuum using the muscles of the neck, shoulders, and upper, mid, and lower back, as well as the anterior chest muscles.

Here's an interesting thought to ponder: When you are training a specific type of muscle in your body, are you actually training the muscle to do the work? If I want to be able to lift weight using the biceps brachii muscle in my arms, and I repetitively do bicep curls with weights, am I training the bicep muscles or am I training the nerve to send signals to the bicep?

We are now understanding through research that repetitive motions and muscle training actually have a greater effect on the signaling nerves than on the muscle itself. The nerves control the signaling to the muscle, thus when we train, we are actually training the nerve to send signals to the muscle more quickly and efficiently than it was previously. The muscle happens to grow because as usage of the muscle increases, blood flow to the area also increases. This blood contains oxygen and macronutrients like amino acids, and it helps to pull out and take away any waste products.

Where you send flow is where you send function.
—Sachin Patel

The important factor to take away from this is that we can train nerves to signal more efficiently and improve their function. In the same respect, if we do not train a specific type of muscle or nerve, the function of that nerve becomes dysfunctional and slow. This less efficient nerve signaling is the first step of nerve dysfunction and dysfunction of a specific nerve and muscle combination.

As for breathing, we have been chronically training ourselves to breathe incorrectly and inefficiently for years for the superficial reasons that have been subconsciously ingrained in each us from early in our lives. This has led to issues in multiple nerves. The phrenic nerve has not been trained to breathe correctly, as we don't generally use our diaphragms to breathe with our bellies. In the same respect, as we are not

Activate your VAGUS NERVE

fully expanding and creating effective vacuum effects, the lungs are not expanding effectively and the vagus nerve signals as such. Vagus nerve signaling becomes less efficient as our breathing becomes less effective.

> *Breathing is the first act of life, and the last. Our very life depends on it. Since we cannot live without breathing it is tragically deplorable to contemplate the millions and millions who have never mastered the art of correct breathing.*
> —Joseph Pilates

Learning to breathe correctly is one of the simplest and best things you can do for your health. Proper breathing techniques are at the root of so many different therapies, practices, and trainings. We will discuss many of these in the next section, which will focus on improving each of these dysfunctions.

Another symptom of incorrect breathing patterns is the inability to control stress levels. Those who feel chronically overwhelmed by emotional and physical stressors often have very poor breathing habits. The next time you get riled up or find yourself in an argument or heated discussion, pause and take a moment to consider your breathing. In these situations, we usually take short and shallow breaths, which activates our fight-or-flight response. Pausing and taking deep breaths helps us become more rational and calm, which helps us create a positive resolution very quickly. Those with poor vagal tone tend not to be able to control their anger, so they will often lash out quickly and raise their voice, altering their breathing patterns toward these shallower and quicker breaths.

Dysfunctional Airways

Remember the last time you had a stuffy nose? Do you remember trying to breathe in through your nose and feeling terrible? At the same time, your energy was low and you likely had a bit of a sore throat or didn't feel great overall. If your airways are not clear, then it can be very hard to breathe in deeply and fully. This can be a constant issue for someone dealing with a deviated septum, chronic adenoid inflammation, and post-nasal drip. All of these issues can lead to the airways not functioning optimally.

Dysfunctional airways are associated with the issue of dysfunctional breathing. When I speak of airways, I am specifically speaking of the nasal passage, the pharynx, the larynx, and the trachea—together, these are known as the upper respiratory tract. There are a few different insults and issues that can affect our airways negatively and I will discuss each one in this section. The first is dysfunctional posture.

We live in the smartphone and laptop age. We sit at our desks and stare at our computer screens for hours on end, then take breaks from our computers to look down at our smartphones. We are all guilty of this, including me. We spend hours in a poor mechanical posture, leading to back and neck pain, then hold our cellphones below our chin. For the most part, we are all aware that postural issues contribute to neck, back, and shoulder pain and mechanical dysfunction of the spine, but it's easy to forget the problems that it causes with airways and the ability to breathe correctly.

Here's another test for you to do right now. I want you to sit in a slouched position. Have you done it? Okay, good.

Activate your VAGUS NERVE

Now, I want you to try to take a deep breath in by expanding your belly—breathe with your diaphragm.

Was it easy or hard? Most people find it more difficult and possibly even painful to take a deep breath in a slouched position. The reason for this is that the middle section of the spine (the thoracic spine) is sitting in a flexed forward position when we slouch. To expand and contract optimally, the diaphragm requires a less flexed position of the thoracic spine and an extended position of the lumbar spine. In a slouched posture, it is actually much easier and less painful to breathe using the accessory muscles.

Another issue when we are looking down at our laptop screens (and even farther down at our cellphones) is that our necks tend to be cranked in a flexed position for longer periods of time. This actually causes us to constrict our airways, so the muscles of the pharynx and larynx are unable to remain tight and allow the airway to stay as open as possible.

This part of the airway is also highly susceptible to weak muscles at another time: during the night, while we are asleep. Snoring and sleep apnea are major health issues and far more common than most people can imagine. During my days as an overweight teenager and in my twenties, I was one of the millions of people suffering from sleep apnea. And like many of these sufferers, my condition went undiagnosed.

Sleep apnea is most commonly caused by some sort of obstruction to the upper respiratory tract during sleep. The most common cause of this issue that I have witnessed in my practice has been vagus nerve dysfunction. Weakness in the tone and strength of the pharynx causes the tongue to collapse toward the back of the throat. This issue tends to affect people that primarily breathe through their mouth rather than their nose. I was one of those people, and I have learned and trained myself to change this habit.

We are meant to breathe through our nose; the mouth is simply a backup plan. After all, our noses have hairs to filter the air, and our mouths have teeth to chew food. Speak to any dentist and they will tell you that without a doubt, the patients who breathe through their mouths have significantly greater oral health concerns than nose breathers. Mouth breathing dries out the saliva and can be considered dangerous. A dry mouth allows bacteria to grow unchecked by antibodies in our saliva, which leads to bad breath (halitosis), tooth decay, and cavities. This issue is also often accompanied by chronic nasal passage obstruction. A lack of airflow through the nasal passage leads to chronic sinus infections and post-nasal drip.

Training yourself to breathe through your nose is possible and will be discussed in greater detail in the next section. It is also important to train the muscles of the pharynx and larynx to increase muscle tone and vagal tone. You can learn to do this by following the recommendations in Chapter 15.

Monotone Voice

A patient suffering from much emotional stress recently came to my office. She had gone through a tough breakup and had some trouble at home with her parents. She was dealing with a diagnosis of irritable bowel syndrome and had been prescribed multiple medications to help manage these symptoms, but with very minimal changes to report from them. One of the signs that I noticed during our initial assessment was that she was not fully capable of increasing and decreasing the pitch and tone of her voice. Her voice was quite monotonous.

Activate your VAGUS NERVE

Monotony is a sign of poor control over the laryngeal muscles, which manage the tension levels of the vocal cords. When someone has a monotone voice, it is a sign that signals are not effectively passing through the motor component of the vagus, thus the muscles are not receiving enough signaling to tense, lengthen, relax, or stretch the vocal cords. This leads to very slight change in the tension of the cords, and thus, inability to control pitch or tone of voice.

I immediately recommended some specific vagus nerve toning exercises to this patient, and in just two months, she was able to notice significant changes in her health and in the tone of her voice. She was able to have greater control of her speech and had improved communication levels with her parents. If you listen closely to yourself or those around you, it is possible to pick up on these small signs that can point you in the right direction.

CHAPTER 6

DYSFUNCTIONAL DIGESTIVE SEQUENCE

Have you been told that you eat too quickly? Have you ever counted the number of times you chew your food with each bite? Next time you eat, take a moment and actually count the number of times you chew each bite of food and how long you actually sit down for your meal.

You may be wondering, "Why does this even matter or make a difference in vagus nerve signaling and your overall health?" Well, the answer is complex, but it makes a lot of sense when you understand the importance of digestive sequencing.

When you get hungry, your brain receives signals from your gut bacteria and from cells in your body, asking to be fed with the required nutrients to create energy and build up reserves for future needs. Each of your cells requires macronutrients.

Fat and carbohydrate are needed primarily for energy production, and dietary protein and its component amino acids are needed for internal protein production. Each of the processes inside of our cells also require micronutrients (vitamins and minerals) to allow these functions to occur. All nutrients enter your body through the digestive tract—but only if the sequence of digestion is adhered to.

My mentor, Sachin Patel, has a great analogy that he uses to explain the importance of the digestive sequence. Imagine you are taking your car to a drive-through car wash. Your car is dirty and you want to get it clean so that it looks nice. You drive to the entrance of the car wash and await your turn to enter. You then drive up to the control panel and punch in your code on the keypad to set up your car wash and indicate that you have purchased a valid option. Only after this code is typed in correctly will the door to the car wash open, allowing you to enter. You then push the transmission into neutral and allow the system to do its job.

As your car is guided along the path inside the car wash, the machines start whizzing and whirring around you. First, your car is misted with some water, followed by a spray of tricolor foaming soap. Rotating cloths brush and spin around to physically activate the soap, form the foaming suds, and push away any dirt attached to the car.

Your car continues to crawl slowly and deliberately toward the next functioning unit. Your car is sprayed down with water once again, this time to remove the soap. As the vehicle continues creeping forward, it passes the air blower, which pushes all the excess water off your car. Upon completing this final task, your car exits the car wash shining, looking as beautiful as it did on the day you bought it.

This process is very deliberate and slow. A specified sequence of events must take place to complete the task and achieve the desired result. This same principle is important for the complete process of digestion.

An optimal digestive sequence takes approximately 16 to 20 hours to complete, from ingestion of food to release of the waste products. There is quite a bit of variation between people, male and female, healthy and unhealthy, but a transit time shorter than 10 hours is considered too fast, while longer than 24 hours is considered too slow. Diarrhea and constipation are very common concerns that 20 to 40 percent of people deal with at any given time. As vagus nerve activation is responsible for digestive sequencing and peristalsis, dysfunctional digestive rhythm is directly correlated to vagus nerve dysfunction.

If digestion occurs too quickly (i.e., in less than 10 hours), you are likely dealing with a lack of nutrient absorption, while digestion taking longer than 24 hours is associated with increased toxin build-up, a rise in opportunistic bacteria, and leaky gut. A longer transit time within the optimal period (16 to 20 hours) is strongly correlated to greater microbial diversity— a healthier and more diverse population of bacteria in the large intestine.

Once your gut bacteria and internal cells decide that they are hungry or in need of nutrients, they send a signal up the vagus nerve to the brain, promoting you to feel the hunger. You are sent to pick up your next snack or meal by the signals sent from your microbiome.

As soon as you see the food, you begin the process of digesting it correctly. If you have ever begun drooling at the sight of a meal that looks or smells delicious, you have experienced this first step. Your mouth is being prepared for the first bite by producing saliva from your salivary glands. Even before you have taken that first bite, your body has already started preparing to break it down. The next step is taking that first bite.

Chewing your food adequately is very important. Your mouth is the only place along the entire digestive tract that has teeth, so is the only place that can physically break down your bite. If you do not chew each bite well enough, then you will not break the food down into small enough morsels to activate the taste buds on your tongue and mouth. The taste of each bite is signaled to the brain to determine how much protein, fat, and carbohydrate is present. Then, the VN signals the stomach, liver, gallbladder, and pancreas to create and pump out the correct amounts of stomach acid, bile, and digestive enzymes. Poor vagus nerve signaling contributes to malnutrition, but this is often overlooked.

You may have noticed that food actually tastes better when you take your time eating, rather than when you are in a rush. This is because you are actually taking the time to chew and send signals up to the brain. People who do this with each meal will actually eat less food than people who eat in a rush, but feel just as satiated and digest their food more readily and appropriately. Eating quickly and not chewing well contributes to a lower level of satiety, higher caloric intake, poorer food choices, and malnutrition.

After chewing, the vagus signals the pharynx and larynx to allow the chewed bite to enter the esophagus and be pushed down to the stomach using peristalsis. Once the food reaches the stomach, stomach acid breaks it down into macronutrients and indigestible fiber. The stomach then continues to churn and push it into the first part of the small intestine. In this location, the liver, gallbladder, and pancreas release their enzymes and bile to help further break down and absorb nutrients into the bloodstream. Upon being absorbed in the bloodstream, fats, carbs, and amino acids are transported to the liver for filtration first, then throughout the rest of the body to be used by the cells for energy production and protein building.

The vagus nerve facilitates movement of the indigestible fiber through the small intestine and ileocecal valve to reach the proximal colon of the large intestine. Here, the large bacterial population breaks down the fiber (which we are unable to process with our digestive enzymes) into vitamins, minerals, and precursors for hormones and neurotransmitters.

The entire digestive sequence is primarily controlled by the vagus nerve, which is constantly signaling to and from the central nervous system and requires a lower level of stress to function optimally. Digestion can only occur in the correct sequence if it is given the right signals from the VN and the proper amount of time for each step to do its part. In the same way that the car wash must receive the correct signals and be given the time to work step-by-step, optimal digestive sequencing and functions require proper signaling and time.

When we grab a quick meal while running out the door in the morning, we are eating in a stressed situation. When we eat our lunches in front of our work computers, we are eating in a stressed environment. When we don't pay attention to the food in front of us, we are unable to send the correct signals to our brain and digestive organs to get the digestive process functioning optimally. Even our dietary choices affect this process and the nerve that controls it.

To optimize digestive sequencing and vagus signaling to and from the digestive tract, it is necessary to have the vast majority of your meals in a low-stress environment. This means taking time to sit down and eating each meal in a relaxed location. If you are at work, go sit outside or at least away from your desk. If you are in a rush, take a cup of coffee or tea rather than food on the go. Even having some papers lying on your dining room table can make the location more stressful and prevent optimized digestive function, because you may be thinking about the fact that you need to clean the house rather than focusing on your meal. Create relaxed, restful environments where you can sit comfortably and eat your meals so you are not beginning the digestive sequence in a stressed state. We will discuss some specific strategies in Part 3.

Bacterial Overgrowth and Vagus Dysfunction

Small intestinal bacterial overgrowth (SIBO) is a common cause of digestive distress. It occurs when the bacteria that should only be in the large intestine overgrow and spread into the small intestine, moving in a backward direction. It is a common cause of IBS, Crohn's, ulcerative colitis, and many other autoimmune conditions. If SIBO is not taken care of with basic herbal and supplement protocols, it can become recurrent.

Vagus activation is necessary to push food forward along the intestinal tract in one direction. If bacteria are moving in the opposite direction, this leads us to understand that there is a weak signal being sent through the vagus that allows this motion to occur. This can happen at the ileocecal valve itself (the valve that stops food from going back from the large intestine into the small intestine) or throughout the digestive tract. For this reason, recurrent SIBO is a common finding when vagus nerve is weak and needs to be activated.

If you are interested to find out about your personal digestive rhythm and bowel transit time, we will discuss the sesame seed test for bowel transit time in Chapter 14.

Dysfunctional Dietary Choices

The single greatest debate regarding our health is what kind of dietary strategy or food plan we should follow. Research does not point to a specific diet as being best for the vagus nerve. The debate over whether we should eat paleo, vegan, ketogenic, pegan, or low-carb is not one I am willing to dive into, as there are many individual factors to take into account, and each diet has positive and negative points.

I will, however, make some recommendations and show you that poor dietary choices can lead to ineffective vagus signaling, dysfunctional digestion, and nutrient deficiencies that affect each cell in the body. Regardless of what diet you choose to follow, some food choices negatively affect our health and are understood to cause issues for a vast majority of people.

Highly processed foods made of low-quality ingredients are the major culprit in this battle. The majority of these foods are found within the aisles of your grocery store. They are the "food products" sitting in boxes and bags in the center of the store, with shelf-lives longer than any of their individual ingredients would last. Foods containing emulsifiers and preservatives to increase their shelf-lives have a direct correlation with increased levels of inflammation and gut microbiome changes toward dysbiosis.

What are these highly processed foods that we should avoid? Most food products with more than four ingredients listed on the package are likely to be poor options. This includes the basics like crackers, breakfast cereals, beverages with added sugar or sweeteners, etc. Low-fat, high-sugar diet foods that claim to be low in calories are often also low in the nutrients your bacteria want and your cells need. Fast food and pre-prepared meals are generally made using low-quality ingredients, which have been shown to increase inflammation and negatively change bacterial populations.

These choices trigger opportunistic bacteria to grow and produce higher amounts of toxins, most commonly LPS, which is known to break down the bonds between the cells of the intestinal tract and enter the bloodstream. This molecule has negative effects on many of our cells, including brain and liver cells. LPS is actually used by researchers around the world to simulate and produce inflammation in their subjects for testing. In high quantities, it produces a life-threatening situation called sepsis, but in chronic exposure to low quantities, as seen in a dysfunctional gut, LPS triggers chronic low-grade inflammation.

Much research shows that activation of the vagus nerve actually reduces the inflammation triggered by LPS. Problems occur as stress levels increase and vagus nerve signaling becomes dysfunctional. This allows LPS to wreak havoc on your gut lining and have far-reaching effects on your immune system, leading to autoimmune disease, metabolic diseases, and even cancers.

Some food choices can reverse LPS-led inflammation and actually help improve the function of the brain, nerves, and even the vagus itself. By volume, the brain is made up of more fat than any other component. The brain and nerves are essentially insulated by fat to ensure their function. In the long term, low-fat diets can actually cause decreased signaling in the brain and individual nerves. The good fats in our diet can improve the insulation around these nerves and trigger proper signaling within the vagus nerve itself. When we take in high-quality, minimally processed dietary fats, our intestines and gut bacteria send a signal of CCK to the enteric nerves and then to the vagus. This activates vagus function and leads to activation of the cholinergic anti-inflammatory pathway.

So what should you eat and what should you avoid? It's a complex question with a very simple solution. As stated by Michael Pollan, the author of the book *In Defense of Food*, the summary is "Eat food, not too much, mostly plants." I take this to mean the following:

- **Eat real food:** Real foods are the things you tend to find on the outer walls of the grocery store, including fruits, vegetables, grains, high-quality seafood, meats, eggs, and poultry.

- **Not too much:** If you eat slowly, you can enjoy each bite and feel fuller while eating less overall.

- **Mostly plants:** About 75 percent of what you eat should grow in or on a plant. Fruits and vegetables are generally unprocessed, contain the vast majority of the nutrients that your body needs, and often taste significantly better than you realize.

Activate your VAGUS NERVE

Our current food choices—heavily processed foods—tend to dissolve very easily, and we don't need to chew them much before swallowing. They stimulate the bad, dysbiotic bacteria that lead to cravings for foods we know we shouldn't eat. These food choices should be rigorously avoided and are one of the major causes of negative health, chronic stress, and disease in the modern world.

Follow one simple rule: Green, Clean, and Lean

I follow this simple rule when I am choosing foods in the grocery store: green, clean, and lean. Green (plants) should make up the majority of your plate and shopping cart. Eat clean foods, meaning unprocessed and organic. And "lean" refers to meats and animal proteins of the highest quality. Healthy fats are also an important component of a good diet, and minimally-processed plant-based fats tend to be the best options. I personally use avocado, olive, or coconut oil to cook with due to their health benefits and minimal processing.

Chemicals on Our Foods

Do you choose organic options whenever possible? If not, you should certainly consider it, if not make it an absolute priority. If you have not heard, the effects of herbicides and pesticides on our health can be significant and have much farther reaching effects than anyone ever anticipated.

Glyphosate is the main culprit here. It is the most widely used herbicide on earth, affecting many of our agricultural crops. The herbicide kills off weeds without actually killing the crop it is sprayed on. Crops such as corn, soy, canola, cotton, alfalfa, and sugar beets are genetically modified to not be affected by the glyphosate molecule. But the glyphosate depletes these crops of a very important micronutrient called manganese, which is required for many functions in our bodies.

The effects of glyphosate and low levels of manganese have been linked to many conditions including anxiety, celiac disease, mitochondrial dysfunction, gout, liver damage affecting bile production, arthritis, osteoporosis, osteomalacia, Parkinson's disease, autoimmune conditions, immune dysregulation, and even infertility. One of the major effects of manganese deficiency caused by glyphosate is high levels of inflammatory activity in the brain. Manganese is required for certain pathways to function in the brain and a deficiency leads to increased immune activation and high levels of inflammatory cytokine release. This is typically mediated by vagus nerve activity, but because brain function begins to decrease, vagus signaling in the brain is limited as well. There are very few mechanisms to slow inflammation in the brain.

Choosing organic food can limit your chances of experiencing the effects of glyphosate. When choosing foods, green, clean, and lean is the way to go. And remember, clean means organic!

Poor Satiety Reflex

I used to have a lot of trouble regulating the amount of food that I ate. I was unable to notice when I felt full near the end of a meal, so I would simply eat and eat. The neurological reflex from my stomach was very slow, and this resulted in my overeating at each meal, as well as having many snacks. This is what led me to become significantly overweight and was the root of my health conditions prior to finding functional medicine.

A poor satiety reflex is one of the most common signs of an impaired vagus nerve in North America today. As we are aware, the obesity epidemic is growing at unprecedented rates. This leads to heart disease, diabetes, and soaring cancer rates. Many of these conditions are preceded by signs of vagus nerve dysfunction, and a poor satiety reflex is one of the most common signs. Whether they recognize it as vagus dysfunction is an entirely different question.

The vagus nerve innervates the stomach and sends information back to the brain regarding the amount the stomach has stretched. Often, it takes time to have this signal completely optimized, and those of us with less than optimal vagus nerve function tend to have an even slower reflex. The inability to feel full or satiated near the end of a meal is a sign that the vagus is not able to send these signals. This issue is exacerbated by the fact that we are living in the fast food era and eating under stressful circumstances. When we do not take the time to rest and digest in the parasympathetic state, it is nearly impossible for us to regulate our food intake, and thus, the vagus nerve is not being exercised and trained to let us know when to stop eating.

Take a moment and think about your stress levels during your last five or six meals. Were you eating in a relaxed environment or at your desk in front of your computer? Were you enjoying a good laugh with loved ones, or were you rushing through the drive-through while trying to make it to an important meeting? The environment in which you eat determines the ability to train your vagus nerve to send these signals to your brain.

CHAPTER 7

DYSFUNCTIONAL MICROBIOME

One of the most likely low-grade stressors that you may not be aware of is the bacteria living in and around you. The population of bacteria living in your gut and on your skin has a significant effect on us, and if that population is not optimally balanced, it can be a major stressor on your body.

In Chapter 3, we discussed the fact that there are approximately 100 trillion bacteria present in our large intestine alone, compared with the 40 to 60 trillion human cells that make up our body. There are even some estimates that state there are 10 times more bacterial cells living in and on us than there are human cells in our bodies. Interestingly, there are 150 times as many genes in our microbiomes than there are in the human genome. It has also been proven that the composition of our microbiomes has a direct relationship to our diet and health as we age.

All disease begins in the gut.
    —Hippocrates

As we know, the vagus nerve is highly involved in signaling to and from the small and large intestines. It signals the digestive tract to activate smooth muscle cells, allowing these muscles to contract. This activates peristalsis following a meal and something called the migrating motor complex between meals. The VN also sends anti-inflammatory signals to the immune cells, ensuring that the system keeps the brakes on as necessary. Information is also relayed from the gut bacteria to the cells of the digestive tract, which then sends signals to the central nervous system via the vagus nerve.

The Effect of Stress on Gut-Brain Function

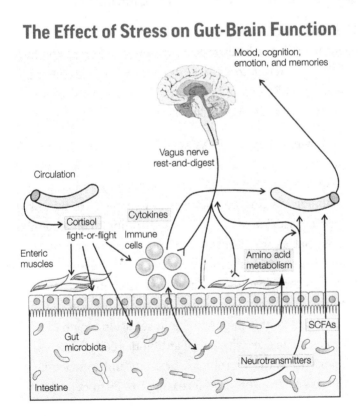

The bacterial population is very important in dictating health and we have learned much about its effects over the last decade. Although we are still unclear about how the VN communicates with the microbiome and which vagal afferents are activated by which gut bacteria, there is much research to show that many of the effects of the gut microbiota on brain function are highly dependent on VN activation and its specific signaling. The byproducts of bacterial metabolism include very important and nourishing molecules called short-chain fatty acids (SCFAs), which are important in reducing the amount of inflammation in the gut and throughout the body. Butyrate is the most-researched SCFA that has shown to be lacking in those with high levels of inflammation.

There has been much research done on what population of bacteria leads to a healthy development and longer life. In *The Psychobiotic Revolution*, the authors summarized the population studies of bacteria based on babies, toddlers, adults, and the elderly to determine what was necessary to be healthy.

Here is what they found as stated by Paul O'Toole and Ian B. Jeffery in "Gut Microbiota and Aging" published in the journal *Science*, "Although not significantly associated with chronological aging, loss of diversity in the core microbiota groups is associated with increased frailty." This essentially means that as we lose microbiome diversity and representation from various groups of bacterial populations, our health suffers, leading to decreased strength and cognitive performance. What we are fed both early and later in life can actually dictate this population and set us on a path of health or disease. The excessive use of antibiotics early in life can significantly skew the microbiome diversity and increase our risk of disease later in life by decreasing the Firmicutes bacteria levels and essentially eliminating Actinobacteria levels. When we have an imbalanced bacterial flora and low microbiome diversity, our levels of SCFAs like butyrate actually decrease, increasing our risk for inflammatory health conditions.

As was discussed previously, the presence of lipopolysaccharide (LPS) can have dramatic effects on ACh receptors. It tends to be high in our bodies due to dysbiosis and poor microbiome balance in the gut. The gene that encodes the nicotinic ACh receptor in humans is highly influenced by the presence of LPS, so it's important to keep these levels low and consistently checked.

Additionally, preliminary studies in mice have shown that the vagus nerve is activated by vagus signaling from specific species of bacteria. A study published in the *Proceedings of the National Academy of Sciences* showed that *Lactobacillus rhamnosus* affected GABA levels in different parts of the brain, improving stress levels and cognition. Notably, this only occurred when subjects had an intact vagus nerve. The researchers suggest these bacterial interactions could be an option for treating anxiety and depression. Another study showed that exposure to *Bifidobacterium longum* can decrease levels of anxiety-like behavior in mice with colitis. The effect was significantly faster and more efficient in mice with an intact vagus nerve. On the other hand, *Campylobacter jejuni* infections can increase anxiety-like behavior—which is linked to inflammation—according to a 2008 study published in *Brain, Behavior, and Immunity*. These reactions were likely activated via the vagal pathway.

The signals that are sent from these bacteria do not interact directly with the vagus, but they send signals through the enteroendocrine cells (EECs), which make up 1 percent of the cells lining the gut. When we eat food, our bacteria interact with that food and send signaling molecules to EECs, which then signal the vagus to increase gut motility, secrete enzymes, and modulate food intake. EECs signal to the vagus directly using serotonin, or through gut hormones like CCK, GLP-1, and peptide YY, as well as ghrelin and orexin. These hormones are important in the signaling of hunger and satiety.

In simpler terms, the byproducts of bacterial breakdown of our food are signaled through 1 percent of our intestinal cells to our vagus, which signals the brain about the activity in the gut. This is why the vagus nerve is so important in cases of obesity and overeating. A less sensitive vagus nerve has been implicated in overeating and feeling less of a reward with a meal. This occurs when the vagus receptors are less sensitive to the stretch of the stomach when food enters, or to the hormones that are released from EECs in the small and large intestine.

Although they make up the vast majority of the microbiome, bacteria are not its only members. It's also important to keep in mind that we may also have viruses, fungi, protozoan parasites, and worms living in our digestive tracts, contributing to the levels of inflammation in our gut. Indeed, there are many parasites that can have functionally detrimental effects on the function of your gut and the signaling to and from the vagus nerve.

A 2015 review by Halliez et al. published in *Frontiers in Cellular Neuroscience* described the effects of certain parasites on the gut: *Cryptosporidium parvum* infections can lead to decreased nutrient absorption due to the parasites breaking down the cells of the gut lining. Abdominal pain is a symptom of a *C. parvum* infection. *Giardia duodenalis* is a parasite that alters gut motility, which has a direct effect on vagus nerve, and prevents nutrient absorption through the breakdown of gut lining cells. Additionally, *G. duodenalis* has a negative impact on the cells in the gut that help produce serotonin, thus potentially reducing serotonin levels. Serotonin is important for signaling from EECs to the vagus nerve as well as regulating your mood. A final example is *Entamoeba histolytica*, which alters cellular function, including electrolyte transportation, secretion, and malabsorption of nutrients, thus affecting the function of all cells, including those of the enteric nervous system, which leads to a direct signaling breakdown to the vagus nerve.

Many other parasites can have significant effects on the function of your gut and the signaling in the nerves, but the important thing to note is that these are blind spots and stressors that are easily overlooked by the conventional medical system. Unfortunately, most doctors have never even heard of many of these parasites, let alone their specific effects on nutrient status, gut motility, and vagus nerve function.

Viruses are also possible causes of nerve dysfunction, as they can enter the body through the gut. There is a very likely hypothesis that viral infection of the vagus nerve itself may contribute to chronic fatigue syndrome. There is a real correlation between poor vagus nerve activity and the symptoms of chronic fatigue syndrome, which include fatigue, sleep changes, loss of appetite, depression, malaise, and cognitive impairment, as well as clinical signs of inflammation and an inability to decrease inflammation.

You can, however, be tested for most of these good and bad members of your microbiome. In my practice, we use a functional stool test called the GI-MAP test from Diagnostic Solutions Laboratory, which uses DNA-PCR technology to identify the specific species of bacteria, parasites, viruses, and fungi that are living in your gut. Using this information, we can determine the correct next steps for eliminating these blind spots that are likely causing significant health issues in those who are dealing with them.

Many of my patients have successfully cleared infections including these parasites, overgrowths of bacteria, yeast, and viruses, which were not discovered as being the root cause of their issues until they came in to see me. This is the power of functional and lifestyle medicine. We will discuss more strategies in Part 3 of the book.

It is clear that the makeup of your gut microbiome has very specific effects on not simply gut function but also on the nerves that signal within the enteric nervous system and along the vagus nerve itself. Balancing the microbial population in your gut is one of the major steps you can take to ensure that the gut is functioning optimally and that vagus nerve signaling is working as it should be.

CHAPTER 8

CHRONIC INFLAMMATION AND IMMUNE ACTIVATION

Chronic inflammation is the most common and obvious sign of ineffective signaling from the vagus nerve. It is unfortunately overlooked by many health care practitioners. Once we are able to test for, determine, and eliminate the root cause of the inflammatory response, inflammation levels should come down. Very commonly, however, these levels do not drop as easily as we would like.

Chronic inflammation can show its face in different ways, from low-grade arthritis-type pain in the knees, ankles, hips, shoulders, and wrists to unmanaged autoimmune conditions that destroy cells without our realizing what they are doing. If the vagus nerve is functioning optimally and can send signals to shut down inflammation levels, then once the cause of the condition has been eliminated, vagus signaling should be able to reduce these levels on its own. Improving vagal tone can help reduce these inflammatory signals and limit the amount of damage they can have on function and structure.

If someone is suffering from chronic inflammation levels that have persisted for months and even years, the first step is to determine and deal with the root cause. As we have discussed, many of our immune and inflammatory cells are housed in the gut. Testing the gut to confirm that there are no inflammatory triggers is the best way to deal with the root cause of inflammation. While dealing with these triggers, vagus nerve tone will help limit the damage, so performing exercises to improve signaling will work effectively to manage inflammatory levels.

Autoimmune Conditions

Do you or someone you know suffer from an autoimmune condition? Autoimmunity is the fastest growing health condition in North America due to our lifestyles, chronic stress, unhealthy diets, and lack of understanding of the true cause of these conditions. I have worked one-on-one with hundreds of patients who have been diagnosed with autoimmune diseases such as type 1 diabetes, multiple sclerosis, Hashimoto's thyroiditis, psoriasis, rheumatoid arthritis, Graves' disease, Crohn's disease, systemic lupus erythematosus, celiac disease, alopecia areata, and many others. The one commonality I have come across is that my patients have not been informed of how the condition started in the first place.

As we now know, the largest volume of our immune cells are located in the gut, in areas of the intestine called gut-associated lymphatic tissue, or GALT. This is where much of our primary immune responses take place, as the digestive tract is quite sensitive to penetration from invaders and toxins. These invaders and toxins are triggers for immune cells to become active, and in some cases, overly active.

Although genetics plays a role in the risk of developing an autoimmune condition, genes are simply a blueprint. The array of environmental triggers are the major reason why these conditions start in the first place. In fact, there is much research showing that genetics determine only one-third of risk of disease development, while non-genetic environmental and triggering factors contribute the remaining two-thirds of the risk.

So what exactly are the factors that determine one's risk for developing an autoimmune condition? In a 2016 review published in *Rheumatology*, Hartmut Wekerle suggests there are three factors that trigger autoimmunity in our bodies:

1. A genetic profile that has risk of developing autoimmunity

2. A certain amount of immune cells (autoreactive T cells) present in the GALT

3. A pro-inflammatory gut microbiome balance

We are not able to change our genes, nor are we able to determine the number of autoreactive immune cells sitting ready for activation in our gut. The only factor that we can affect at this time is the microbiome—the balance of gut bacteria, parasites, viruses, and yeast that trigger or slow inflammation based on the signals it sends our cells. The vast majority of signals from the microbiome are healthy. But when we don't feed our microbiome correctly, the population can change and allow pro-inflammatory bacteria and other opportunistic gut bugs to take over. An imbalance activates the immune system, increases inflammation, and triggers the autoreactive immune cells in the GALT.

Chronic Inflammation of the Gut

Do you remember the analogy of the police and the immune system in the gut? The autoreactive immune cells—the immune cells that monitor the function of our human cells—are these police officer cells. High levels of inflammatory signals over a longer period of time will have a negative influence on policing cell function and will cause autoimmune conditions if the correct factors are present.

How can we find out if we have chronic inflammation levels in our gut? The stool test that I use in my office (GI-MAP DNA stool analysis from Diagnostic Solutions Laboratory) is great at telling us exactly what is living there—any potential autoimmune-triggering bacteria that send out these high inflammatory signals, as well as the current level of immune system function and the amount of inflammation in the gut.

There are other sources of inflammation besides gut bacterial imbalances, but microbiome imbalance is by far the most common that we see in our office. An inflammatory diet full of highly processed, low-quality foods is another very common reason for these signals to arise.

As we are aware, the effect of the vagus nerve is to slow the level of inflammation and keep it in check. If we are sending repeated messages of inflammation over a long time, we are essentially training the vagus nerve to stop having its positive anti-inflammatory effect. This is why it is most common for people to begin experiencing and receiving diagnoses of these autoimmune conditions in their 30s and 40s. After 30+ years of inflammatory signals, the vagus nerve has been trained to stop functioning as an anti-inflammatory intervention. Between the ages of 35 and 40, the vagus tone has decreased significantly and the anti-inflammatory signals stop being sent out. These conditions often arise following the stress of pregnancy, having children, and lacking sleep during the first years of a child's life—all of which are stressors that decrease vagus nerve function.

Inflammation Due to Physical and Emotional Trauma

My patient, Shelley, suffered from symptoms of severe anxiety, heart palpitations, and hormonal acne, as well as deep concerns about her increasing weight. She had gone through multiple episodes of high stress in her life: Both of her parents had passed away from cancer only two years apart, and her brother and sister-in-law had both passed away three weeks apart in severe and tragic events. Her health was suffering and her symptoms worsened through each of her two pregnancies. Her hormones were a mess, her mindset was negative, and she was not happy at all. She was dealing with a mass of emotional and biochemical stress.

Inflammation is a protective mechanism that occurs in our bodies to protect us from damage; it does not only increase in response to biochemical signals from the gut. When a child bumps their head or falls down, they may develop swelling or a bruise in a localized area, which is actually a collection of cells and cell signals working to repair any damaged tissue. Problems tend to occur when signals for inflammation take place over a longer timeline. Inflammation levels are good for the body, but only if they are kept in check by the vagus nerve and the cholinergic anti-inflammatory pathway.

Repetitive signals for inflammation due to physical trauma can occur for various reasons—multiple automobile accidents, multiple pregnancies, repetitive strain injuries, improper weight-lifting technique, and weaker muscles are all possible sources of chronic physical injury and inflammatory signaling.

Emotional trauma can include stressful life events that create a negative impact on one's mindset. These are especially effective if they happen in succession during a short period of time. Life events such as the passing of a loved one, the loss of one's job or income, emotional and mental abuse, or the emotional burden of a severe physical injury impacting independence are common and seen by functional medicine doctors like myself quite commonly in practice. Traumatic life events that we have trouble overcoming have the ability to put us into the fight-or-flight state, which amplifies the inflammatory process. If we then experience a small physical trauma, inflammation levels are easily increased, leading to chronic inflammatory processes that are difficult to keep under control. Emotional trauma may not be the trigger for inflammation to occur, but it enables a state that amplifies the effect of physical trauma.

Often a single event of physical trauma can be the inciting event to push our inflammation levels over the limit, instigating symptoms of other diseases and conditions to show themselves. Patients often explain that their autoimmune

Activate your VAGUS NERVE

condition seemed to start following pregnancy and delivery of their children, or even following a small car accident. In these cases, the most likely scenario is that inflammatory signals were barely under control by the VN, but this single event caused inflammation levels to spike and bypassed the amount that VN had been trained to handle. Thus, the inflammatory signals amplified, and symptoms began to appear more readily in the weeks and months that followed that single event.

A high incidence of these traumatic events will certainly take a toll on the body. In Shelley's case, her body and mind had gone through multiple severe stressors in a relatively short time. Once we were able to organize her thoughts and get her stressors and hormones balanced, she progressed significantly, and in just five months, she saw significant improvements in her hormonal health, weight levels, and overall happiness. With our guidance and by working on her microbiome and vagus nerve signaling, she was able to improve her health and decrease the amount of stressors her body was negatively experiencing.

CHAPTER 9

DYSFUNCTIONAL HEART RATE

We are told that the average resting human heart rate is between 60 and 100 beats per minute. The more calm and collected you are, the lower the heart rate will be, and the more stressed out you are, the faster your heart will beat. Electrical signals from the vagus nerve and sympathetic nerves dictate change to the heart rate. The lower your resting heart rate, the stronger your vagus nerve. Interestingly, there are studies suggesting that one's lifespan is inversely correlated to resting heart rate—thus, the lower your heart rate, the longer you will live. From this, we can extrapolate that stronger vagus nerve tone and function is associated with lower heart rate and thus a longer natural life expectancy.

When a car goes spinning out of control on an icy road, the driver will immediately feel stressed and enter the fight-or-flight state. The sympathetic nerves activate immediately and the vagus is shut down. The signals from the sympathetic nerves speed up the heart rate by signaling that the muscles of the arms and legs need much more oxygenated blood to control the steering wheel and push on the brakes of the car.

Once the car comes to a safe stop, the sympathetic nerves slowly stop firing and the vagus is able to turn back on. The effect of vagus is to slow the heart rate using calming, rhythmic electrical signaling.

One sign of a dysfunctional vagus nerve is the inability to quickly normalize the heart rate after this type of stressful event. The amount of time a person spends with a high heart rate and shallow breathing following a stressful occurrence is a strong sign of vagus nerve function. One who is able to quickly calm their nerves and slow their heart rate has a very strong vagus nerve, while someone who takes longer to come back to their resting rate is likely suffering from dysfunctional vagus nerve tone. How well do you function under the pressure of a high-stress situation like this? Do you remain very calm and rational when dealing with such a scenario?

The opposite of this issue—an uncontrolled, overactive vagus—can also occur. Vasovagal syncope is a major issue caused by underactive sympathetic nerves and a hyperactive vagus nerve. Syncope is the medical term for fainting. The sympathetic nervous system acts to increase heart rate and blood pressure while the parasympathetic nerves act on the heart to slow heart rate and decrease blood pressure. If the sympathetic nerves are weak and the vagus nerves are overactive, the result is a temporary loss of consciousness that is not life-threatening.

This condition can manifest in otherwise healthy individuals and have devastating immediate effects. Though there is no indication of long-term effects, vasovagal syncope is a sign of improper balance within the autonomic nervous system. It is a common concern without a single clear cause. In fact, there are many different causes, and the mechanisms are very different between younger and older individuals.

The most common theory is that the imbalance of sympathetic to parasympathetic activity is triggered through a physical head tilt motion, such as sitting or standing quickly after lying down. This postural change leads to a change in blood pooling location, from within the chest to within the abdomen, and in turn, the heart muscle struggles to maintain its pumping activity. With the change in the amount of blood being pumped out of the heart comes a significant change in blood pressure. The autonomic nerves work to maintain a safe blood pressure, but if they are unable to do so, blood pressure drops suddenly, which takes place immediately before the episode occurs. Once the body is given a moment to regulate the blood pressure, the individual can regain consciousness and will feel fatigued or nauseated due to the changes that occurred.

Although this mechanism points to a physical trigger for the fainting episode to occur, it does not speak to why the autonomic system is unable to regulate the heart and blood vessels to ensure a safe change in posture. This is a type of dysautonomia, or the decreased ability to regulate autonomic activity. The mechanisms that lead to dysautonomia can be genetic, as with Charcot-Marie-Tooth disease and Ehlers-Danlos syndrome, or they can physically manifest, as with pregnancy, physical trauma, chiari malformations, or surgery. The most common causes, however, are related to immune and metabolic health conditions. When the cells of the nervous system lack the correct nutrients for healthy metabolic responses or are dealing with high levels of toxicity in the body, the nerves are not able to function quickly enough. Even more of a concern are autoimmune conditions that affect the nerves themselves, as well as the organs innervated by the VN and the sympathetics. These conditions include Parkinson's disease, sarcoidosis, Crohn's disease, ulcerative colitis, Sjogren's syndrome, amyloidosis, and even chronic inflammatory demyelinating polyneuropathy.

When someone deals with an issue like vasovagal syncope and has relatively common fainting spells, it is often a sign of an immune or metabolic issue that may not yet be diagnosed. Functional lab testing and functional neurology provide insights to the potential underlying root causes of this issue, which is often a symptom of improperly functioning nerves in the autonomic nervous system and hyperactivation of the vagus. Changes in heart rate, blood pressure, and cardiac output that cannot be fully regulated are signs that vagus and the autonomic nervous system are not functioning optimally.

CHAPTER 10

DYSFUNCTIONAL LIVER FUNCTION

Your liver performs hundreds of tasks every second. From continuously sensing and managing blood sugar to filtering toxins from the blood to producing bile salts, the effects are far-reaching and affect the entire body. The liver requires a certain set of nutrients to do its job optimally, just as a professional chef in a five-star restaurant requires his or her preferred tools, like high-quality knives and cookware, otherwise the job will not be done to the highest possible standards.

One of the liver's jobs is to detoxify the blood, essentially filtering out any hormones, neurotransmitters, drugs, and toxins that should not be present in high quantities. Toxins can be produced inside the body as end products of metabolism or as endotoxins, which are released by bacteria and cross into the bloodstream. They can also be exotoxins such as drugs, agricultural chemicals, food additives, household chemicals, and pollutants. These toxins can be either fat soluble or water soluble. The liver has a two-stage filtering process that it uses to clear all of these potentially harmful substances out of the blood.

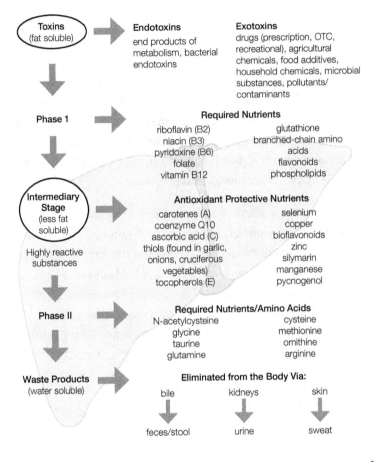

Toxins (fat soluble)

Endotoxins
end products of metabolism, bacterial endotoxins

Exotoxins
drugs (prescription, OTC, recreational), agricultural chemicals, food additives, household chemicals, microbial substances, pollutants/contaminants

Phase 1

Required Nutrients
riboflavin (B2)
niacin (B3)
pyridoxine (B6)
folate
vitamin B12
glutathione
branched-chain amino acids
flavonoids
phospholipids

Intermediary Stage (less fat soluble)

Antioxidant Protective Nutrients
carotenes (A)
coenzyme Q10
ascorbic acid (C)
thiols (found in garlic, onions, cruciferous vegetables)
tocopherols (E)
selenium
copper
bioflavonoids
zinc
silymarin
manganese
pycnogenol

Highly reactive substances

Phase II

Required Nutrients/Amino Acids
N-acetylcysteine
glycine
taurine
glutamine
cysteine
methionine
ornithine
arginine

Waste Products (water soluble)

Eliminated from the Body Via:
bile — feces/stool
kidneys — urine
skin — sweat

In the first phase of detoxification, five different types of reactions occur so the fat-soluble toxins can become less fat soluble. These reactions require many B vitamins (specifically B2, B3, B6, and B12), folate, glutathione (one of the strongest antioxidants in the body), branched-chain amino acids, flavonoids, and phospholipids. Many of the patients that come to see me are deficient in most of these nutrients, either because their diets are lacking these nutrients, or because their digestive processes are not effectively getting these nutrients into the body.

Once the liver completes the first stage, the toxic substances tend to be highly reactive and are a risk to the health of our cells. These highly reactive substances are called reactive oxygen species, and we need a strong set of functioning antioxidants to counter any damage they may do to our cell surfaces and even our DNA. These antioxidants include vitamins A, C, and E, coenzyme Q10, thiols, selenium, copper, bioflavonoids, zinc, silymarin, manganese, and pycnogenol.

If the liver has enough nutrients (including many of those required for phase one), these reactive oxygen species undergo the six reactions of phase two to become entirely water soluble. One of the reactions is called amino acid conjugation, and it requires certain amino acids—N-acetylcysteine, glycine, taurine, glutamine, cysteine, ornithine, arginine and methionine. The end products of this process are water-soluble toxins that can be released via urine, sweat, and stool.

It is essential that the liver have access to all of these nutrients, as well as enough energy-producing fats and carbs, to fulfill its tasks on an ongoing basis. Otherwise, toxins are essentially free to roam the body and cause harm to any cells they deem fit, leading to high levels of protective inflammation. Remember that the VN is essential for ensuring inflammation does not become chronic and have deleterious effects.

In functional medicine, liver function, including detoxification, is absolutely imperative and one of the first things we

Activate your VAGUS NERVE

look to correct when beginning a protocol with a patient. By showing the levels of specific metabolites secreted in the urine, organic acid testing can give a clear indication of liver function and detoxification processes. Before we attack and rebalance any gut bacteria, we must ensure that detoxification processes are working well. If not, the body is likely suffering from a low-grade chronic inflammatory process that can negate the effects of the vagus nerve over time.

A strongly dysfunctional liver will often lead to fatty liver, which is becoming a much more common diagnosis, as well as an enlarged liver (hepatomegaly) and even potentially cirrhosis of the liver. It is important to remember that the liver is the fastest regenerating organ in the body. Given the correct nutrients, a poorly functioning liver can recover quite quickly and begin functioning optimally to perform its many tasks.

CHAPTER 11

CHRONIC STRESS

Imagine that you are in the gym working out and lifting weights. You are holding a long barbell that you are lifting repetitively from the shoulder to overhead positions. There is some weight on each side of the bar, but it is very manageable. You feel good while doing it, as you know that this is a good stress on your body. You are training your nerves and muscles to be able to lift this weight over your head, and you feel a greater sense of accomplishment with each lift that you successfully perform.

Now imagine that someone comes by and adds an extra 20 pounds on each side of the bar. The weight is still within what you can manage to lift, but it's starting to get quite heavy. Then, someone else comes by and adds another 10 pounds on each side of the bar. You begin to struggle lifting the bar overhead. They add another 10 pounds, then another 10 pounds. You are seriously struggling to lift this weight, and even just holding it is quite difficult at this point. You are sweating, shaking, and worried that you are going to drop the bar and potentially hurt yourself. Finally, someone comes and helps you by taking off the last 20 pounds from each side. The weight has become manageable once again. As your stress levels increase, your ability to handle the stressors increases, but the load can become too heavy if it is not kept in check.

In this analogy, the weight on the bar represents the stressors in your life. We all must experience some good stress to grow. Yes, I said good stress, also referred to as "eustress." These are challenges that help us to grow and feel our best. Some common types of eustress include working out at the gym; traveling to experience a new part of the world; having a baby and helping it to grow into a healthy, happy adult; and a new romantic relationship and the beautiful stressors that come along with this experience. These are all positive stressors that our bodies are able to lift relatively easily and repetitively from shoulder to overhead positions.

Occasionally, though, external stressors come along and add extra weight to our bar. These can be negative stressors, which are commonly called "distress." Some common types of distress include financial stress, poor communication in a relationship, health concerns, and the death of a loved one. These stressors can be perceived negatively and cause us to feel burdened by the weight we are lifting overhead. It may be necessary, and in many cases advisable, to seek external support to help take some of this weight off the bar.

The difference between positive and negative stressors is not that one is inherently building you up while the other is knocking you down. Rather, the difference comes from your perception of the stress and the effect that it is having on you. This may be a little philosophical, but keep it in mind, as it is a very important factor in your health. If you believe that a stressor is positive, then it will have a positive effect, while if you believe that a stressor is negative, it will have that effect on you.

Parking your car far away from the entrance of a store or mall has exactly this effect. If you believe that it is negative and that you are being burdened by the long walk ahead of you, the perception is negative and it will affect your mood as such. On the contrary, if you feel that the long walk is an opportunity for you to get some more steps in your day and enjoy a bit of exercise, then it will have a positive effect on your mood and health. If you are interested in reading deeper into this, I highly recommend a book by Dr. Bruce Lipton called *The Biology of Belief.*

Consider that we are not always aware of all the stressors in our lives. We may be suffering from excess weight on the bar and not even realize that it is present. Somehow the weight that we are carrying feels heavier than it looks. In the case of your health, the stressors that are placed on your bar are often invisible, burdening you with weight you are unaware of. Many of these are caused by habits that we have and may not realize. I call these "lifestyle habits" and the good news is that once you become aware of them, you can change them. However, if you are unaware of them, they can add extra stress to your body. We will discuss these stressors in more detail soon.

Our bodies handle all types of stress, whether good or bad, in the exact same way. We shift from a comfortable rest-and-digest state to a fight-or-flight state, in which we are able to either stand up and battle the stressor or run away from it. The body will react the same way to negative financial stress and positive gym workout stress, undergoing the exact same process as our evolutionary predecessors who had to handle the stress of running from a pack of saber-toothed tigers and starting fires.

In the fight-or-flight state, we begin to sweat, shake, and send blood flow away from the rest-and-digest organs toward the muscles of the arms and legs. In the rest-and-digest state, the vagus nerve signals for blood flow to increase toward the digestive organs and the parts of the brain that make you feel rested.

These states are not binary. Fight-or-flight vs. rest-and-digest is not like a switch that you can flip to turn a light on or off. It is actually a continuum.

For our bodies to function optimally, we should be on the parasympathetic side of this continuum the vast majority of the time. In other words, the weight that we are carrying on the barbell should be very manageable. We should be able to carry it easily and function well internally. Approximately 80 percent of the time, we should be activating our vagus nerve and remaining in a relatively parasympathetic state.

It is important, however, that we can quickly and easily shift toward the sympathetic state to manage stressors that may arise at any moment. We tend to be able to do this quite easily thanks to the neurotransmitter adrenaline and hormone cortisol.

We make the jump to a high-grade sympathetic state when an immediate stressor occurs. Imagine what your bodily response would be when you get into a car accident, or when somebody jumps out from behind a door to scare you. You immediately get scared and get into a defensive mode. Your heart begins to race, your eyelids blink, but then you open your eyes wide to see everything that is happening around you. You begin to take short, fast breaths and may start sweating right away.

To imagine the parasympathetic state, you can picture how you feel when you are on vacation, lying on the beach, listening to the ocean waves crashing nearby. Your body is relaxed, feeling like it is able to digest correctly, sleep correctly, and recover from any stressors that may arise. It should not be a surprise to you at all that you feel so much better and healthier when you are on vacation.

Health issues begin to occur when we have trouble switching back from the sympathetic state to the parasympathetic state. When the weight that we are lifting is very heavy and we are having trouble managing it, then it is tough for us to switch back toward the calmer, easier rest-and-digest state.

This common scenario involves the constant burden of stressors and the belief that the stressors are negative. When we remain in this state, we tend to turn off vagus nerve activity; we stop training it. We instead increase the activity of our sympathetic nerves in a chronic, long-term way with continual exposure to low-grade stressors. If this continues for a long time, we will slowly decrease vagus nerve tone and lean toward vagus nerve dysfunction.

What are these chronic low-grade stressors that I speak of? These are the stressors of the daily grind—sitting in traffic on the way to work, going in to work each day at a job you may not love, worrying about the meal that you and your family are going to have each night when you haven't planned in advance, etc. There are so many mild little stressors that add two, three, and even five pounds to the bar you are carrying, and although the weight of each stressor is minimal and not very heavy, the sum of all these small weights is much heavier than we realize. These stressors cause an imbalance in our hypothalamic-pituitary-adrenal (HPA) axis function, which can inhibit our ability to manage energy and stress levels throughout the day.

It's not stress that kills us, it is our reaction to it.
—Hans Selye

If your body is burdened by chronic low-grade stress the majority of the time, then you will not be able to activate the necessary processes of the vagus nerve. Over time, this low-grade sympathetic state will lead to decreased parasympathetic activity, which yields increased inflammation, decreased immune cell activity, poor digestive function, less effective detoxification, and many other problems that can cause health issues. This is exactly why most people who are suffering with health concerns tend to deal with multiple health conditions throughout their lives. These are conditions that affect multiple organs and the health of each one of our cells.

One of the most important factors in your health will be your ability to bring yourself back to a parasympathetic state from a sympathetic state. Patients that tend to get better faster and experience amazing results are the ones that learn to create positive lifestyle habits so they can more quickly, efficiently, and readily shift their state from sympathetic back to parasympathetic. To be able to make changes in stress levels, we must first be able to identify all of the stressors that our bodies may be under, especially the invisible stressors that are taking place in our blind spots. The strategies that my patients use to identify their stressors and create positive changes are discussed in Part 3 of the book.

Chronic Stress

It's not the load that breaks you down, it's the way you carry it.

—Lou Holtz

Inability to Handle Stressful Situations

In an interview with a friend and colleague of mine, Dr. Jared Seigler, we discussed many of the common signs of vagus nerve dysfunction. Dr. Seigler spoke about patients that have come in to see him for an assessment, and these people are dealing with high vagus nerve function and a complete burn-out of the sympathetics. These people often have significant issues handling stressful situations. They have trouble with large crowds, loud noises, and tight spaces. This is an autonomic dysfunction, caused by the vestibular canals being unable to suppress their emotional response.

If your sympathetic neurons are weak, then keeping an emotional balance will be very tough, especially in these situations. These patients are also often dealing with issues with their balance, as the vestibular system is linked to autonomic function and control of emotions; they also can have greater volumes of tears from the lacrimal glands and saliva production from the salivary glands in the mouth.

These are signs of imbalanced autonomic function, skewed toward sympathetic weakness and parasympathetic dominance. It is possible to recreate these symptoms in patients with basic vestibular testing such as head tilt exercises or spinning around in a chair. These movements can elicit

Activate your VAGUS NERVE

significant changes in heart rate and breath rate and lead to digestive slowing.

As we discussed earlier, the strength of the brain is based on the strength of the nerves. To determine how strong the vagus nerve really is, we must test it against a baseline and come up with the best way to ensure this system is actually working. Testing methods will be discussed in Chapter 14.

CHAPTER 12

DYSFUNCTIONAL SLEEP AND CIRCADIAN RHYTHM

How well do you sleep? Do you wake up feeling rested and full of energy in the morning? When we sleep, we go through five cyclical stages of brain activity. Stages one and two are lighter sleep, often associated with the first 7 to 15 minutes of falling asleep. Stages three and four are the deep restorative sleep stages that are associated with muscle and tissue repair, growth and development, boosted immune function, and production of energy for the next day—essentially, all of the tasks mediated by the vagus nerve to help our bodies perform at their best the next day. Vagus nerve activity (measured through heart rate variability) has been shown to be significantly higher during stages three and four of sleep.

The fifth stage is rapid-eye movement (REM) sleep. During this phase, heart rate variability decreases. It has been shown that parasympathetic activity significantly decreases during this phase of sleep. Sympathetic activity predominates REM sleep, which is associated with formation of memories as well as dreaming.

These phases will take place at different times of the night as we age, but in adulthood, the first four stages are more likely to be cyclical and occur earlier at night, while REM is more common later in sleep. This is why so many people wake up during a dream and are able to recollect specific moments of that dream. We will normally run through five to six cycles of REM sleep each night, which also means we enter the deep restorative sleep about the same number of times.

Deep restorative sleep is the gym for the vagus nerve.

The vagus nerve trains during deep restorative sleep, stages three and four of the sleep cycle. Just as a weightlifter will train a specific group of muscles or a yogi will train their body to perform postures, the VN must train to function at its best. This means that if you are not getting a good, restful sleep at night, you likely are not entering the deep restorative stages required for vagus training—thus, you are not training the vagus nerve. As with most other nerves, if you don't use it, you lose it. However, I prefer a different quote regarding nerves: If you don't train it, you drain it (of the ability to perform optimally). Training your nerves is highly important to their function, and just as getting to the gym is important in training the nerves that activate your muscles, deep restorative sleep is a gym for the vagus nerve.

Getting to bed at an optimal time is essential for allowing the vagus nerve to train. Guidelines tell us that optimally, we need eight hours of sleep each night.

Do you eat meals or snacks late at night? Relatively recent research shows that vagus nerve afferent fibers actually express clock genes in the nodose ganglia. This essentially means that the vagus nerve acts as a peripheral clock based on the amount of food present in the stomach. There are certain times when sensitivity to stomach expansion is high and certain times when sensitivity is low. If you have ever felt like you ate too much, too late at night, it's happening because the stomach is significantly less sensitive to stretching during the night, when the sun has gone down. If you are going to sleep at a late hour, eating meals late at night, and feeling drowsy or lacking energy early the next morning, your vagus nerve is likely firing at inopportune times, leading to dysfunctional nerve firing.

It is important to not only choose the right foods, but to eat them when there is still light out and you are awake to properly digest this food. The sensitivity of the stomach decreases at night, so we are more likely to overeat later in the evening than we are during the late afternoon and early evening.

Activate your VAGUS NERVE

CHAPTER 13

LACK OF SOCIAL INTERACTION

We need to be around people. Face-to-face social interaction is supremely important for our health. If you've ever spent a few days at home, alone, I'm sure you started to feel a little down and moody. Well, this isn't just some off-the-cuff feeling that you are having. It turns out that your vagus nerve is actually activated when you are in a social situation and interacting with people face-to-face.

My mentor, Sachin Patel, pointed out to me that in prison, the punishment for doing something wrong is to be put in solitary confinement—literally being placed in a small box by yourself, with no interaction for hours and even days on end. We would rather be surrounded by other convicted criminals including murderers than be in a cell, all alone.

A 2009 study by Schwerdtfeger et al. in *Health Psychology* showed that heart rate variability—a great way to measure vagal tone—decreases in those with less social interaction and a depressed mood. Symptoms of depression are found to be associated with a lack of vagal tone. When patients with these same symptoms were put into social situations, their mood, heart rate variability, and autonomic control of the heart increased—namely, vagus nerve activity.

This finding was reinforced by a study in *Biological Psychology*, by Kok et al., just one year later. Adults recruited from a university had their vagal tone measured at the beginning of the program and again nine weeks later. Individuals with higher vagal tone scores predictably had greater increases in feelings of connectedness and positive emotions. Even more importantly, these individuals actually saw an increase in vagal tone at the end of the study.

Depression is directly linked to low vagal tone.

These studies show that our feelings of happiness and positivity are directly connected to vagus nerve activity and vagal tone. Those with higher vagal nerve activity actually feel more positive and experience social interaction in a more positive light. Depression and low mood are directly correlated to lower levels of vagus nerve activity.

This means that the more positive, in-person social interactions you have, the more you train your vagus nerve to function optimally. People who live in isolated environments with limited social interaction are not able to train their vagus nerves to their greatest ability and are more likely to suffer from health conditions caused by inflammation levels that cannot be controlled by the VN. Positive emotions build physical health while negative emotions lead to physical dysfunction and disease.

Activate your VAGUS NERVE

PART 3

ACTIVATING YOUR VAGUS NERVE

CHAPTER 14

MEASURING VAGUS NERVE FUNCTION

Anything that can be measured, can be changed.

In functional medicine, we have a saying that we hold close and promise to practice with: We don't guess—we test. Determining vagus nerve function is no exception to this. We may base many of our recommendations on the symptoms that a patient presents with, but there is no replacement for an objective test that tells us the best steps to take for each individual patient.

In this chapter, I will discuss the four methods we use to measure vagus nerve function and determine if the VN is functioning optimally or needs training. These methods are the measurement of heart rate variability, heart rate, breath pattern, and bowel transit time. The most important thing to keep in mind is that anything that can be measured can be changed. If you test your vagus nerve function and it is currently not optimal, you will be able to activate it and optimize its function if you personally make the effort to do so.

Heart Rate Variability

Heart rate variability (HRV) is the gold standard for measuring vagus nerve function. No single test is considered a stronger and more accurate representation of the activity levels of the vagus nerve and vagal tone. It is measured most accurately in a laboratory setting using very expensive and sophisticated equipment; however, with a reasonable investment, we can measure it at home with a good amount of accuracy.

Remember that the vagus nerve has the effect of slowing and regulating the heart rate to a comfortable resting pace. There are four chambers in the heart: the left and right atria, through which the blood enters the heart; and the left and right ventricles, which pump the blood into the blood vessels so it can make its way around the rest of the body.

The "lub-dup" of a beating heart actually represents the two phases of the heartbeat. The first pump of the heart—the "lub" portion—represents the action of the muscular walls of left and right atria, pumping blood into the ventricles. The "dup" portion is much stronger; this phase represents the thicker ventricular walls pumping blood into the aorta and pulmonary artery, sending oxygenated blood to the cells of the body and deoxygenated blood to the lungs. Following the "lub-dup," there is a short period of time called an "interbeat interval" during which there is no electrical activity expected to take place in the heart.

Heart rate variability is the measurement of time, in milliseconds, between successive pumps of the heart—the time from the end of one "lub-dup" to the beginning of the next "lub-dup." Whether and how much the time between pumps varies is an important indicator of both cardiovascular and autonomic health. The more active your vagus nerve, the lower your heart rate will be, within an optimal zone, and the more variable the time will be between pumps of your heart.

If your heart did not have any parasympathetic or sympathetic nerves innervating it, it would pump at approximately 100 beats per minute (bpm). Sympathetic innervation could elevate the heart rate to 120 bpm. A heart rate around 120 bpm is quite high and means that there are approximately two heart beats taking place each second. This means that there will be approximately 400 to 450 milliseconds of time between each pump of your heart. One would consider this as low HRV, as the time between pumps remains relatively constant—the variation between beats is 38 milliseconds at most.

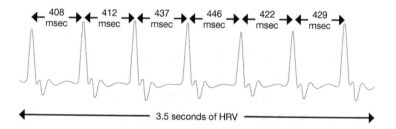

Parasympathetic innervation, on the other hand, helps lower the heart rate and increase heart rate variability. Once the heart rate drops down to its normal resting state, HRV can be measured to determine just how healthy a person truly is and how well their vagus nerve is firing. Optimal heart rate is between 50 and 70 bpm, and HRV should be significantly

Activate your VAGUS NERVE

varied between each pump. This would be considered an example of high heart rate variability, as there are 130 milliseconds of variation between beats. The higher your heart rate variability, the more likely you are to have a higher level of fitness, cardiovascular health, and vagal tone. High HRV is also one of the best predictors of longevity.

As technology improves and becomes available to the general public, tools emerge allowing us to take control of our health and by measuring these health predictors on our own. There are two tools I personally use and encourage my patients to use as well.

The first tool I use is the Inner Balance tool from HeartMath. It is a great basic tool for anyone interested in learning about their heart rate variability and overall health, while also wanting to take steps to improve their HRV. The Inner Balance tool teaches you to improve your heart rhythm and send positive signals of health and longevity to the brain via the vagus nerve. The goal of HeartMath and the Inner Balance tool is to enter a state called coherence and to increase your HRV with regular training. When we are in a state of coherence, our HRV is high and our bodies are functioning in an optimal state.

The great thing about this tool is that it can be used with your smartphone. It will connect with Apple or Android to relay information to you about your current level of function and coherence. It can teach anyone to enter the state of coherence, which is extremely valuable in high-stress situations, especially for those who tend to be in a chronically sympathetic state.

There are all types of new and upcoming wearable technology, many of which are meant to monitor how your body is functioning. The most important thing to consider when deciding how to track your performance is whether you may be exposed to electromagnetic radiation or other suboptimal energy fields, and to what degree. More and more data shows that exposure to different types of radiation have less than ideal effects on one's health. Many of my colleagues and I use the Oura Ring because, when using it in airplane mode, it limits exposure to dangerous electromagnetic frequencies (EMF). Once I remove it from my body, I can share the data with my phone.

Oura Ring tracks interbeat intervals using a technique called photoplethysmography. The best part about the Oura Ring is that you can wear it all the time and it gives you real-time data for your full day, as opposed to just when you attach a tracking unit. The Oura Ring can track your current state, your recovery from endurance or training exercises, your readiness to perform a new exercise, drops in activity that may signal an oncoming infection or cold (even before you get symptoms), sleep quality, how your body handles stress, and even whether you are dehydrated (which can lead to a drop in HRV). (If you decide to buy one, visit OURAring.com and use the special code "vagus" to get a discount on your purchase.)

Resting Heart Rate and Heart Rate Recovery

Resting heart rate is a simple measurement that tells you how well your body is functioning. If we consider that average resting heart rate is generally between 60 and 100 bpm, but without any autonomic stimulation the heart rate would be approximately 100 bpm, it is safe to extrapolate that the

Activate your VAGUS NERVE

lower your heart rate within the optimal range, the stronger the parasympathetic signaling to the heart.

Optimal heart rate in a healthy individual should be in the region of 50 to 70 bpm. Many athletic individuals tend to find their heart rate on the lower end, 50 to 60 bpm, while less active but still healthy individuals will tend to have a heart rate of 60 to 70 bpm. New research shows that a resting heart rate above 76 bpm is linked to an increased risk of heart attack. In fact, the risk of dying from any cause is correlated to an increase in heart rate in both men and women. Essentially, as resting heart rate goes up, the higher the chance of dying from any cause, especially one that is cardiovascular.

After exercise, it is important to measure how quickly your heart rate recovers to its resting rate. High-intensity exercise and training is known to lower resting heart rate over time, and consistent training is linked to faster recovery times. If it takes you a long time to recover following an exercise session, this is a sign of poor cardiovascular health and poor vagal tone; remember, vagus signaling is necessary to slow heart rate and maintain resting heart rate. Optimal recovery from exercise involves a drop of 12 bpm each minute, while unhealthy individuals take longer and tend to have a decrease of less than 12 bpm.

To measure heart rate recovery, check your resting heart rate a few times while relaxed. You can use a smartphone or wearable technology to get a relatively accurate finding and record this number. Then, perform your normal exercise or training routine and immediately test your heart rate at the end of the session, using the same method as earlier. Test again after 2 minutes, 4 minutes, and 6 minutes. After 2 minutes, your heart rate should drop by more than 24 bpm, after 4 minutes by more than 48 bpm, and after 6 minutes, it should be very close to your original resting heart rate. This is, of course, dependent on how rigorous your training was and if it was aerobic (e.g., running) or anaerobic (e.g., weight lifting).

If you are tracking your heart rate and HRV regularly, you will notice an increase in HRV following exercise; your vagus nerve is highly active during the recovery process as it works to repair tissues. If aerobic and anaerobic training exercises and tones the muscles, heart, and spinal nerves, then recovery is the training session for the vagus nerve. The more you train, the more you recover, and the more effectively your vagus nerve will fire the next time you exercise. This is why recovery rates improve for those who exercise regularly: The VN is training to perform its job with greater effectiveness and tone.

Paradoxical Breathing Pattern Test

Are you using your diaphragm to initiate your breath? Have your breathing patterns become irregular and caused your vagus nerve to function less than optimally? This is a very simple test and a tool that you can use to train yourself to breathe with your diaphragm.

Sit straight up in a chair or lie down with your back on the floor. Place your right hand on the center of your chest and place your left hand on the center of your belly. Now take a deep breath in. If your right hand is moving more than your left hand, then you are breathing incorrectly. During the inhalation phase, our bellies should be rising and falling more than our chest is, so if we are breathing correctly, our left hand should be rising and falling more than our right hand.

Activate your VAGUS NERVE

Many people will find that their chest is moving more than their belly. This is a sign of paradoxical breathing and shows that someone is likely not using their diaphragm to breathe fully, deeply and correctly. If you are breathing paradoxically, don't worry, because you can train yourself to become an effective breather once again. It will simply take some effort and a daily practice to re-learn patterns that you had long ago when you were a child. See page 132 for breathing exercises.

Sesame Seed Bowel Transit Time Test

How well is your digestive tract moving food? Is it moving at an optimal, healthy pace? As we discussed in Chapter 6, we need our food to be processed and broken down on a specific timeline for our bodies to receive the important nutrients that come from our food. The sesame seed bowel transit time test can give us some information about how our digestive tract is functioning and if we need to make some changes to our health. All you will need for this test are one tablespoon of golden or yellow sesame seeds, one cup of water, a watch or clock, and a notepad and a pen.

We know that our gut lacks the enzymes to digest and break down sesame seeds (similar to corn), which is what makes them so effective for this test. We also know that the vagus nerve is the driving force for peristalsis and keeps the digestive tract moving at an optimal pace. Any variations from this pace can signal a loss of VN control or some other digestive dysfunction.

Here's how to do the test. First, add the sesame seeds to the cup of water and stir it around. Next, drink the cup of water with sesame seeds in it, being sure to not chew the seeds. Take a look at the time and mark it down on your notepad or in your phone. Then, wait until the next time you need to go to the bathroom for a bowel movement. Each time you go to the bathroom and have a bowel movement, take a look and see if you notice any sesame seeds in your stools. Mark down the times and continue checking until you no longer see any seeds. The optimal time in which to see the seeds begin appearing is around 12 hours after ingestion and the latest is around 20 hours after. Seeing seeds 16 hours after ingestion indicates optimal digestive sequence and function.

If your body is pushing the seeds out very quickly, your digestive tract is not working hard enough and the VN is likely not firing optimally. If your body is very slow to eliminate the seeds, then vagus activity is certainly decreased. In either case, testing of the gut microbiome is highly recommended, as it can uncover the cause of poor bowel transit time and potentially poor vagus nerve signaling.

***

Now that we understand some simple ways to measure VN activity and to determine just how well our parasympathetic nervous system is firing, we can get into the exercises and tasks that improve the function of this nerve and help to balance the cardiovascular, respiratory, immune, digestive, and detoxification systems of our bodies.

Activate your VAGUS NERVE

CHAPTER 15

EXERCISES TO ACTIVATE THE VAGUS NERVE

In this chapter, I will dive into each of the active exercises and practices that you can undertake to activate your vagus nerve without purchasing expensive equipment. Much of the research on this topic shows that active exercises performed regularly are as effective as (if not even more effective than) purchasing tools to stimulate the VN. You can find a summary of daily protocols, as well as weekly and monthly goals, starting on page 173.

The practices and exercises discussed in this chapter are all found to be effective at increasing vagal tone. It is important to remember that the vagus nerve is not simply a parasympathetic signaling nerve: The VN has four separate components, each of which can be stimulated to allow optimal signaling and activation of the other three components. These components are:

1. skin sensation from the central section of the ear;

2. motor innervation of the pharynx and larynx;

3. parasympathetic innervation of the heart, lungs, and other organs; and

4. afferent vagus neurons that send signals back to the brain through visceral fibers.

Keep these four components in mind as we go through these exercise options.

Breathing Exercises

The first and most effective way to positively affect your vagus nerve is to learn to breathe correctly. Simply put, rapid, shallow, chest breathing is a sign of stress, which activates the sympathetic branch, while slow, deep, belly breathing is a sign of rest, which activates the vagus nerve.

Breath is our one window into the autonomics.
—Dr. Jared Seigler

The vast majority of us have not learned to breathe correctly. In fact, we have subconsciously trained ourselves to forget the correct mechanics of breathing. If you haven't yet completed the paradoxical breathing pattern test on page 128, I highly recommend doing it now. Correct breathing patterns are directly linked to autonomic nervous system function and altered breathing patterns tell the body that it is under stress.

Activate your VAGUS NERVE

This fact is even more amplified once you realize that the average person takes approximately 23,040 breaths per day.

When we want to learn the best, most efficient, and most effective way to breathe, we must look toward leaders and examples that live amongst us. Consider some of the greatest vocal and instrumental performers of our time. If you have ever attended a concert or opera, you have likely noticed that exceptional singers and instrumentalists can sing an entire set of songs without much of a break. In songs recorded by greats such as Frank Sinatra, Aretha Franklin, and Celine Dion, the artists rarely sound as though they are out of breath or unable to hold a note because they trained their breathing patterns. Opera singers are some of the most effective breathers on the planet; they have learned to control the function of their diaphragm while holding the vibration of their vocal muscles.

Another group to consider are high-performing professional athletes. These are the best of the best—those who do not crumble under pressure. Stars like Michael Jordan, Tom Brady, Cristiano Ronaldo, Tiger Woods, Wayne Gretzky, Nolan Ryan, Ken Griffey Jr., and Babe Ruth all had one thing in common—they were all able to control their stress levels by ensuring that their breath patterns stayed optimal while they were performing. To perform at such high levels, these performers trained themselves to remain calm under high-stress circumstances by using a slow, calm, and comfortable breathing pattern. You, too, can learn to create an optimal breathing pattern that can signal to your body that you are not under stress, thus allowing optimal signaling via the vagus nerve and parasympathetic nervous system.

Multiple research studies have shown that slow breathing exercises are highly effective in improving heart rate variability. One study showed that slowing your breath rate to six full breaths per minute for five minutes was effective in increasing HRV immediately. If this is individualized, the effect on HRV is even more effective. Determining the slow breath rate that is optimal and feels right for you individually will have the greatest positive effect on your HRV levels.

Here are simple steps to practice this exercise:

1. Sit up straight without allowing your back to rest against anything.

2. Exhale completely to remove all air from your lungs.

3. Put your right hand on your chest and your left hand on your belly, just above your belly button.

4. Take a deep breath in through your nose for five to seven seconds, allowing only your belly to rise (feeling only your left hand rising).

5. Hold that breath for two to three seconds.

6. Exhale through your mouth for six to eight seconds, allowing your belly to fall (feeling only your left hand falling).

7. Hold your breath, without any air entering your lungs, for two to three seconds.

8. Repeat steps 4 through 7 as many times as you feel comfortable or for a set period of time.

Take five minutes per day to practice deep belly breathing on your own and your body will thank you. For best results, perform this practice multiple times per day, especially during periods of stress. Even a single minute of concentrated focus on slow, deep breathing can have significant positive effects on your mood, stress levels, and overall health. Work to focus your attention on breathing in through your nose rather than your mouth to make this exercise even more effective when you are practicing it.

If you have already learned to practice this simple deep breathing exercise and are up for something a little more challenging and advanced, I recommend trying the Wim Hof breathing exercise. Wim Hof is a Dutch "daredevil" according to Google, however in learning his method, I now see him as a visionary. He is also known as the "Ice Man" as his training and methodology involves the use of breathing exercises and cold exposure as well as commitment to the practice. To learn more about the method and to take his free online mini-course, please check out his website www.wimhofmethod.com.

Breathing Patterns During Sleep

Now that we have discussed the importance of optimal breathing patterns when you are awake, it's time to ask: What about when you are asleep? The average person requires between seven to eight hours of restful sleep per night, during which they take approximately 7,200 breaths. This is important, as nearly one-third of our breaths are taken while we are not awake. We can train ourselves to breathe optimally when we are conscious and in control of our actions, but what about when we are asleep?

Research has shown that we tend to fall back to poor breathing habits while we are asleep. This is important because obstructions of the airways can affect our health and bodily function negatively when we are not fully conscious. Obstructive sleep apnea is a growing problem and must be addressed if we want to improve our health. I have personally dealt with sleep apnea and know that many of you are also experiencing symptoms, though you may not realize that it is happening. I was only made aware of the issue once I got married. My wife pointed out to me that I would stop breathing in the middle of the night without any reason and I was also snoring quite severely. This was negatively affecting my sleep, and as you can imagine, it sent a stress signal to my body, as it was essentially choking multiple times during the night. Additionally, it indicated that my vagus nerve was not functioning optimally. The symptoms improved when I eliminated much of my excess body fat, but they still popped up from time to time, especially when I was extremely tired before falling asleep. It was an issue until I learned a great tool from a colleague and friend of mine, Mike Mutzel, and Dr. Mark Burhenne, DDS, who was a guest on Mike's podcast High Intensity Health. This tool is called mouth taping and I now use it all the time.

Like me, Mike was dealing with a mild case of sleep apnea. On the podcast, Dr. Burhenne spoke about this great tool and all the benefits it has. When we stop breathing through our nose, we immediately begin using our mouth to breath. Over time, the loss of airflow through the nasal passage has negative effects on nasal microbiome and the cells lining the nasal passage. This leads to obstruction of these nasal passages, post-nasal drip, and increased histamine responses, such as seasonal allergies.

Mouth taping involves putting a piece of tape over your mouth to seal your lips while you are asleep. This essentially forces the airflow to go through your nose while you are asleep. No single tool has been more effective in improving my breathing

Activate your VAGUS NERVE

patterns, allowing me to get a deeper, more restful sleep, and decreasing my allergies.

When we breathe through our mouth, it is far more difficult to use the diaphragm to breathe, but when we breathe through our nose, it is entirely second nature and habitual. HRV studies have shown that we improve vagus nerve function when we breathe through our noses versus pathologically through our mouths. Active breathing exercises during the day and mouth taping at night are a strong combination of tools that one can use to improve their breathing patterns both during the day and at night.

Getting Great Sleep

We all know the importance of getting a good night's rest. Here, I will give you some tools that you can use as part of a bedtime routine to increase the chances of a healthy, restful night of sleep. A restful night of sleep has been shown to improve autonomic balance through heart rate variability studies.

Eliminate Blue Light Exposure in the Evenings

Light wavelengths change throughout the day, and our bodies have adapted to their signals. When the sun rises in the morning, light is quite warm, in the red/yellow wavelengths. By noon, the light is much more blue and sharp. Once again, in the evenings, when the sun is setting, the light turns toward a red/yellow hue. These are the signals that our body uses to tell us the current time of day, as well as which hormones and signals to secrete at precise times.

Our screens, including the laptop, TV, phone, and tablet, all emit a blue wavelength of light. If we look at our screens each evening right before bed, we send a signal to our bodies that the time is actually noon. This will slow the release of melatonin, an important hormone required to help us relax and fall asleep soundly. Some devices now come with built-in blue-light filters, but most do not.

To reduce blue light exposure while still using devices and screens during the evenings, you can:

- Enable Night Shift on your Apple devices

- Download the Twilight app on Android devices

- Download f.lux or Iris on your computer (Mac or Windows)

- Use blue-blocking sunglasses if you are watching the television

For blue-blocking glasses, I recommend using the TrueDark Twilight sunglasses, which are the gold standard of blue-light blocking technology.

Instead of looking at your screen at night, I recommend reading a physical book or spending device-free time with loved ones or friends, as social connectedness is another great way to improve vagus nerve function.

Shut Off Electronics at Night

One of the best things I have ever done for my health was to cancel my cable TV subscription. It forced me to stop watching TV at night. I have since taken steps to reduce electronic

Activate your VAGUS NERVE

use in the evenings and nights, and get noticeably better sleep having done so.

Charging your devices such as cell phone or tablet in a different room, shutting off Wi-Fi routers with an automatic timer, and even putting your devices on flight mode are great ways to stop using them in the evening.

Don't Eat or Drink Too Late

Nighttime bathroom breaks commonly break up restful sleep. If you eat or drink later in the evening, then you are preparing your body to need to use the washroom at night. Instead, have your final meal at least two hours before you sleep and your last drink of water at least one hour before bedtime. Your waistline and your energy levels will thank you the next day!

Love Your Space

Sleeping in a clean, organized space is imperative to improving your sleep quality and your health. When your bedroom is a mess, you can't help but go to sleep thinking about the cleaning and organizing that needs to be done. This negative energy creeps into your mind and makes your sleep restless, which is simply added stress on the body and an easy way to turn off the parasympathetic recovery system at night.

Have a feng shui assessment done on your space to ensure it is organized in an energy-positive way to help you feel great and allow you to grow. Ensure that you clean and organize your space regularly, as this has a direct effect on your mood and energy levels. I recommend reading *The Life-Changing Magic of Tidying Up* by Marie Kondo to learn more about how a clean space transforms the energy in your body.

Sleeping on Your Side

A 2008 study by Yang et al. published in *Circulation Journal* compared the HRV levels of different sleep positions. The study was done to determine the best position for patients dealing with coronary artery disease compared to those without any blockages in their coronary arteries. The researchers found lying on your back is the worst position for HRV levels, both for test and control patients, while lying on either side showed significant improvement in HRV levels. Most interestingly, sleeping on the right side was found to be the best for vagal modulation, especially in the control group.

What this essentially means is that sleeping on your back, or lying on your back for a longer period of time, will have negative effects on vagus nerve function, while lying on either side (right side preferred) will actually allow you to increase vagus nerve tone. This is because when you are lying on your back, your airway is more likely to close, as your tongue can fall backward due to the pull of gravity. This is not nearly as easy when you are lying on your side. Remember, an open airway is absolutely essential for control of breathing, both in terms of breath rate and depth of breath.

To make it easier to sleep on your side, I recommend placing a pillow between your knees while you sleep. This will force you to stay on your side while you are asleep and will not allow you to shift to sleeping on your back.

Cold Exposure

Have you ever jumped into a lake or pool, only to realize that the water is frigid and freezing you to your core? Your teeth begin chattering and your body begins to shiver uncontrollably. Your breath is completely out of your control as well. You take extremely shallow breaths and are unable to rest your diaphragm enough to calm down and breathe deeply.

As you can imagine, this scenario is great for activating your sympathetic nervous system and the fight-or-flight response. Your body is fighting to survive in the short-term, and this has an immediate effect on how your body reacts. Your breath becomes shallow and rapid, your heart rate increases, and your body does not desire to digest optimally during this time. All this short-term effort is meant for survival.

What you may be surprised to hear is that this actually has the amazing effect of activating the parasympathetic nervous system in the long-term. Continuous acute exposure to cold, or cryotherapy, teaches you to regulate your breath, which has an overall positive effect on vagus activation and significant anti-inflammatory effects throughout the body.

Periodic cold exposure is one of the best and easiest ways to activate and heal a lost vagus nerve. The simplest way to incorporate this into your life is to add cold exposure to your showers. One great tip I give to many of my patients is to take a normal shower, then at the end of the shower, turn the temperature down to as cold as possible and let it hit you on your head and the back of your neck for the final minute of your shower. It will initially be shocking to your system and will change the way you breathe. Your goal during this time is to work on controlling your breath and taking as many deep belly breaths as possible. If you can train your body to breathe through the cold, your vagus nerve will become very strong and your body will have an optimally functioning parasympathetic nervous system and vagus nerve. As this minute becomes easier, you can add one or two minutes per week of cold exposure until your entire shower is spent in ice-cold water and there is a huge smile on your face!

Cryotherapy is an emerging and proven science that is used to help reduce inflammation and activate healing via the parasympathetic nervous system. The vast majority of professional athletes, as well as performers such as Tony Robbins, use cryotherapy following each game or performance. Mr. Robbins swears by it for his own health and has found it to have significant healing benefits.

Even Wim Hof, the creator of the Wim Hof method, incorporates cold exposure into this method for its amazing healing benefits. He is known as the Iceman, as he regularly engages in ice baths with his clients and teaches about the benefits of cold exposure. If you feel that cold showers have become redundant and too easy, try going out for a hike on a mountainside in just a pair of shorts and boots. A Google image search for Wim will show him doing just that.

Humming or Chanting

Another way to activate your vagus nerve is to stimulate and use the voluntary muscles that it signals. By activating these muscles, you stimulate the brainstem centers that send signals through the vagus—not just the muscle control centers, but all the others around it as well.

By humming and chanting, you can activate the laryngeal muscles, which get signals directly from the superior and recurrent laryngeal branches of the VN. They allow our vocal cords to tighten and loosen based on muscle tension, thus giving us a level of pitch in our voices. When we practice humming deep in our throat, we are activating and vibrating these muscles and stimulating vagus to send these signals.

Perhaps you are aware of the sacred Hindu syllable "om" that is used to create a deep vibration in the throat when recited out loud. The vibration of "om," which is said to vibrate at the resonance level of god, has a strong spiritual affiliation in the practice of Hinduism. In other cultures, simple words are used such as Amin, Ameen, and Amen; however, they seem to all mean the word of god.

In the vagus nerve, vibrating at this frequency by chanting the word actually stimulates the laryngeal muscles of the throat and vocal cords, allowing stimulation of the motor fibers of the VN. If done for long enough and with enough strength, it can be a strong method of stimulating the other signaling components of the nerve. It allows us to control our breath, slow down our thoughts, and center ourselves to the point of extremely deep relaxation, and has been shown to improve digestion and inflammation levels in the body. Humming or chanting the word "Om" prior to a meal can be a great way to calm yourself down, align with the universe, and stimulate vagus nerve activity to the digestive tract and other visceral organs. Practicing "om" during other times, including following a stressful event, is a valuable tool in decreasing stress levels and sympathetic activation following this stressful event.

There are other words to hum or chant that can actively stimulate these muscles and improve vagus nerve signaling, but "om" is one that I have personally found to be highly effective, as the vibration of the throat muscles is highly evident during the practice.

Activating Gag Reflex

Along the same lines as humming and chanting, activation of the gag reflex is another way to stimulate the muscles innervated by the VN. Also known as the pharyngeal reflex, this reflex, which involves a loop of nerve activation to work optimally, is required to protect us from choking.

When an object that we are not aware of enters our mouth and touches our soft palate (the soft part at the back of the roof of your mouth), a very fast sensory signal is sent through the ninth cranial nerve, up to the brainstem, and to the motor aspect of three different cranial nerves. The first of these nerves is the pharyngeal branch of the vagus, which immediately contracts the three pharyngeal muscles at the back of the throat to stop the object from entering the body farther and potentially getting stuck in the airway. Cranial nerve five and cranial nerve twelve are also stimulated and cause the jaw to open and the tongue to thrust forward to push the object out.

Voluntarily activating the gag reflex will send an immediate signal to the vagus and the other nerves to keep them signaling quickly and optimally. The best time to do this is twice per day, while you are brushing your teeth. You can use the toothbrush to touch the soft palate and stimulate this reflex. This is a great and simple option that is known to have a direct effect on the signaling of VN. As we have a set of cranial nerves on either side of our body, stimulating the soft palate on both sides is necessary to receive the full benefit of this exercise.

Activate your VAGUS NERVE

Gargling

When I was a child, my father often encouraged me to gargle with salt water after brushing my teeth in the morning and evening, just as he has practiced every day for his entire life. He used to tell me that it was good for my health—yet I would laugh it off and make light of this advice. Interestingly, he was on to something. I should have known; he is a very healthy septuagenarian.

Gargling is the act of holding a sip of water in the back of your throat and swishing it around with vigor. It requires activation of the three pharyngeal muscles at the back of the throat, and as such, it is another method of stimulating the vagus nerve through muscle activation. As my father would consistently remind me, practicing this twice per day after brushing teeth is a great way to easily harness this tool.

For best results, gargling with extra vigor, to the point where your eyes begin to form tears, is optimal. When your vagus is firing, it actively sends signals from its brainstem nuclei that activate some adjacent nuclei as they get stronger. In this case, the superior salivary nucleus is being stimulated, which triggers the glands around your eyes to produce fluid that becomes tears. If you are gargling hard enough to make yourself tear, you are doing this correctly and having a great effect on your vagus nerve.

Adding some salt, such as Himalayan pink salt, to the water you are using to gargle is also a great option. Gargling salt water has been shown to have antibacterial effects and can help eliminate some unwanted bacteria from the mouth and upper respiratory tract. Using essential oils, such as oil of oregano, in your water is another great option with very similar effects.

Yoga or Pilates

Yoga and Pilates are not meant to just exercise the body, but to calm the mind and regulate the breath. These methods exercise optimal voluntary breath regulation while increasing external stressors and teaching you how to control your breath.

Most yoga sessions are bookended with a slow deep belly breathing exercise. The idea is to teach you to maintain your breath pattern while your body is held in various different positions. Each of these positions engages the body with a different type of physical stressor. To increase the level of stress within this practice, we have learned to use heat and humidity, which are even more engaging. Moksha and Bikram yoga are two examples of this.

If we can learn to maintain a slow, deep belly breath during times of stress, our bodies are able to function at much greater levels. If we train ourselves to handle voluntary stressors by maintaining our breath, then we can be trained to maintain composure and handle other stressors with significant ease.

Pilates was created as a practice around learning to breathe correctly. We have discussed this requirement much earlier in the book but it is absolutely critical to our health. If we are breathing paradoxically during periods of low stress, our bodies will not be able to handle periods of high stress.

Both yoga and Pilates, when taught with a focus on the breath, are great tools for optimizing breathing patterns, improving

Activate your VAGUS NERVE

inflammatory responses, and activating the VN to function optimally.

Mindfulness Practice

Prior to starting a task, do you take a moment to sit still, close your eyes, and focus your attention? Do you ensure that you are putting 100 percent of yourself into the task at hand? When you are resting, do you take a moment to become grateful for your surroundings?

Mindfulness is exactly this: taking the time and making the effort to pay attention to what you are doing and what is happening around you. Many of us jump from task to task, or put out one fire after another without paying attention to what is going on around us. We get so caught up in our own minds that paying attention to a single task and giving it our full attention gets put on the backburner; it feels like a waste of time and effort to do this.

Many health care professionals, myself included, are guilty of this. We go from patient to patient or appointment to appointment, forgetting or not giving our full attention to the fact that someone is trusting us with decisions involving their health and their life. Becoming a functional medicine doctor has allowed me the opportunity to affect the lives of my patients in a positive and deep way, and as such, I am far more conscious of the attention I can give each of my patients. Prior to bringing in my next patient, I take a couple of minutes to review my notes, remove any distractions from my vicinity, and clear up tasks involving other things. Once I do that, I take a moment to remember that each patient trusts me to help them achieve their goals in health and in life.

Mindfulness practice means performing each task to your greatest capability with 100 percent of your attention directed at that task. It means taking in your surroundings, being aware of everything that has brought you into that exact moment, and being grateful for it.

The ability to practice mindfulness cannot occur when we are stressed out, inflamed, and in pain. Our sympathetic nervous system tends to hijack our attention and prevent us from focusing on what we are doing. If you actively practice mindfulness throughout the day, you are focusing on your breath and how you can achieve each task at hand. This shifts the balance toward the parasympathetic nervous system and allows the VN to do its job.

Approaching a task mindfully means doing one thing at a time with full attention and finishing it before moving on to the next task. Eating mindfully allows you to feel satiated and not overeat. Mindful relaxation allows you to feel rested and rejuvenated sooner than you'd imagine. All of these require the vagus nerve to be active and engaged, as we must be able to rely on so our bodies can rest, digest, and recover. Multitasking is exactly the opposite of mindfulness.

Becoming mindful of what I am doing, eating, and feeling as each task approaches has been the most positive change I have made in my life, and it is by far the number one reason my health outlook became more positive. It has been a major needle-mover for me and for countless others around me, and I'm certain that it can make profound positive changes in your life as well.

Meditation

Meditation is similar to the practice of mindfulness. It is the art of paying attention to your breath and teaching your attention to not follow each thought that pops into your mind. Our brains are designed to think and form dynamic, ingenious connections between our thoughts and actions. Meditation teaches us to listen to our hearts and focus on our breath, learning to become observers of our thoughts rather than victims of their fluidity.

Rather than debate the countless methods of meditation, I want to discuss its benefits. Heart rate variability studies have shown that meditation has significant positive benefits on vagus nerve function because as we meditate, our attention moves toward our breath. There are many different types of meditation but those that are focused on the breath are typically best for improving HRV levels. These include breathing meditation, loving-kindness meditation, vipassana, and mindfulness meditation.

One interesting tidbit of information I found through my research is that HRV only showed improvement in patients who did not label themselves as perfectionists. In the *International Journal of Psychophysiology*, a study by Azam et al. found that control patients were far more likely to have positive changes in HRV levels compared with those who self-identified as perfectionists. Essentially, "perfectionists" were so focused on meditating perfectly or in the correct way that they didn't allow themselves to relax and benefit from the practice itself. One of the most common things I hear when I ask my patients about meditation is that they are "not able to do it correctly." This perfectionist attitude is exactly what is stopping them from realizing the benefits. When practicing meditation without any expectations or preconceived notions about "the correct way" to do it, it is easier to benefit from the practice.

For beginners, I recommend using guided audio meditations found on YouTube or through an app on your phone. I recommend Headspace, Oprah Winfrey and Deepak Chopra's 21-day meditation experience, Calm, and Insight Timer. For those who want feedback on the meditation practice, HeartMath's Inner Balance is a great tool to help you determine if you entered a state of congruence, which is measured through heart rate variability. Another tool for those interested in getting direct information is Muse, the meditation headband, which measures brainwave activity and gives you real-time audio feedback. These are add-on tools and are not at all necessary to practice, but they can be a good investment for those who typically strive toward perfection.

Laughter and Social Connectedness

If you knew that laughing more would improve your health, would you do it more often? Remember the last time you had a good laughing session with friends. Did you feel great for the next few hours? Did you sleep better that night? Did you wake up feeling great the next morning?

Ongoing research repeatedly shows laughter and laughter yoga to be very effective in improving mood and heart rate variability. We tend to use our diaphragms when we laugh with vigor and enjoyment, and in turn, we exercise our ability to control our breath rate and ensure we can normalize our breathing patterns. This is exercise for the vagus nerve.

Activate your VAGUS NERVE

Making vigorous laughter a regular occurrence is a great and very enjoyable way of improving vagus nerve function. I make a point of watching funny videos or going to comedy shows as often as possible to feel connected socially, and to enjoy the health benefits of laughter. Taking laughing yoga classes in your community, meeting with friends regularly to exchange fun stories, and turning on a comedy movie are all great options to laugh more. Social connectedness is directly involved with this, as we are more likely to laugh out loud when we are in the presence of others, especially friends and family. Social connectedness is one of the greatest determinants of health and can be even more important than the food you eat.

People want to be around other people. When we feel lonely and disconnected from others, our mood and health are both negatively affected. We tend to enjoy the company of others and prefer having conversations with real people, face-to-face. When we are around others, we tend to laugh more, smile more, and feel more relaxed.

We feel even better when we spend time with people we resonate and share values with. I was recently able to take my family to a Living Proof Team Retreat in Minnesota, which was an amazing experience. The beautiful natural environment and surroundings were coupled with spending time with team members that share the same values that I do. We were taken care of by the team at Point Retreats, another spectacular group of individuals that values bringing people back to healthier and happier lives. At the end of the trip, we were all very happy and relaxed, regardless of the stress of travel.

If you are feeling lonely, down, or simply disconnected, find a way to spend time with others and connect to people with similar values to yourself. If physical fitness is an important value, join a gym or attend a yoga class with friends. If communication is an important value to you, then join a toastmasters group and practice your public speaking skills with supportive, like-minded individuals. If you value quality time with others, then go to a movie or a meal with friends so you can converse and have a great time. There are 7 billion people on the planet and countless activities and interactions that allow you to connect to these people.

It is believed that as we age, we laugh less, but the healthiest people I know make a point of laughing more. And in the blue zones, the regions around the world with the highest rates of longevity (with many people living past 100 while still being physically active), social connectedness is a common theme.

So get out, enjoy social experiences with those around you, meet new people, exchange fun stories, and laugh as loud and as often as you can. Doctor's orders!

Listening to Music

Don't you feel really good after listening to some great music and singing along? This is because your body is actually feeling relaxed and is able to perform recovery processes during and after this time. It's the same reason why we love to belt out the lyrics to our favorite tunes while sitting in our cars or stuck in traffic.

A 2010 study by Chuang et al. showed that cancer patients who participated in a 2-hour music therapy session that included singing, listening, learning, and performing music showed significant increases in heart rate variability measures, and thus in vagus nerve and parasympathetic nerve activity. Another study by Lin et al. in 2014 used HRV to show that Mozart's music can improve parasympathetic nerve function. Much of this research has been completed with children diagnosed with epilepsy, a common seizure disorder. Listening to Mozart's music, especially Mozart's "K.448" sonata for two pianos, showed a decrease in seizure recurrence and brain changes.

Next time you are sitting in traffic and feeling stressed that you are late for a meeting or for work, turn on some good music and let your body move and sing along with it. You will inevitably feel more relaxed and less stressed, and you will still get to your meeting at the same time. If you are at home and feeling out of it, play Mozart in the background and notice how you feel after.

Music has healing power. It has the ability to take people out of themselves for a few hours.
—Elton John

Smart Dietary Choices

As the research is slowly becoming clearer, we are discovering that there are foods that can have a negative impact on our cellular and digestive health and which have a higher likelihood of increasing inflammation levels. As discussed in Chapter 6, most of these choices are highly processed foods; foods that are contaminated with antibiotics, hormones, herbicides, and pesticides; and foods that are genetically modified. Avoiding these foods is critical in reducing the risk of damage to the gut lining, liver detoxification system, and health of each of our cells.

When choosing healthy and smart foods, I recommend organic, locally grown fruits and vegetables; lean, free-range chickens and eggs; lean, grass-fed and grass-finished beef; non-GMO grains like rice and quinoa; and organic nuts and seeds. For a majority of people, a green, clean, and lean diet made with healthy fats and minimally processed food is the best place to start. To learn more about dietary options, I recommend reading *Food: What the Heck Should I Eat?* by Dr. Mark Hyman. Follow his protocol for four weeks, then reintroduce one food at a time. Remember, your diet needs to be individualized to your needs and preferences. Vegan, autoimmune paleo, paleo, and ketogenic diets are all helpful, but a diet should be suited to what you need. Remember that green, clean, and lean are my personal three rules when shopping at the grocery store or farmer's market.

When looking to specifically increase vagus nerve function, foods that contain nutrients helpful to the production of ACh are essential. Acetylcholine is the major neurotransmitter used by VN, and low levels can contribute to suboptimal vagus nerve activity and signaling. Nutrients that are necessary to allow ACh production are high in choline, such as egg yolks; high-quality cooked organ meats like beef, chicken, and turkey livers; and soy lecithin, a common food additive.

Another effective tool to use in improving vagus nerve function is to give it a rest—literally, let your vagus nerve take some time off. Intermittent fasting and time-restricted eating are effective tools in improving heart rate variability. This is a tool I personally use to balance blood sugar, improve energy levels, and limit the amount of stress on my body. Intermittent fasting has been shown to increase HRV, a sign that vagus nerve function is optimized and health is improving over the long term.

To do intermittent fasting or time-restricted eating, limit food intake to a six- to eight-hour window while you are awake. For example, you can limit calorie intake at breakfast time, thus limiting the amount of sugar present in the blood early in the day, and have your first meal at lunch. I personally eat two meals each day, between noon and 8:00 pm, while taking an amino acid powder each morning to ensure that my cells have the tools they need to function optimally. To learn more about this practice and try it yourself for a 2-week period, join my online Energy Boost Challenge at www.energyboostchallenge .com.

Daily Movement or Exercise

Our bodies are built to move. Muscles are some of the most important and most overlooked organs of the body, and muscle cells are the best at helping us balance our blood sugar and body fat levels—if we use them. The issue is that the majority of us sit and lack movement for a very long time each day, and then we sit in the car, and sit on the couch, and repeat this lack of movement on a daily basis.

Practicing some level of movement, preferably one that helps increase your heart rate by increasing bodily stress levels for a short period of time, helps improve parasympathetic nerve activity. There are times when both the sympathetic and parasympathetic systems can be activated, and post-exercise recovery is one of these circumstances. During the recovery state, we are optimizing our breathing pattern, which increases signaling to the muscles of the airway to increase patency, trains the heart to become stronger and pump out more blood with each pump, and allows us to shift back to a parasympathetic state on a regular basis.

Moving your muscles and getting your body to do things that stress it out on a daily basis will teach the body how to recover from the stress more quickly, while also helping you balance energy levels and macronutrient fuel sources. Use your muscles to make your body do things, preferably outdoors.

Sunlight Exposure

Exposure to sunlight throughout the day is directly linked to your sleep. Our bodies are genetically programmed to work based on the amount and type of sunlight that enters our eyes and skin. It has a direct effect on how we function on a cellular level. If we spend an entire day indoors under artificial lighting with limited exposure to true sunlight, we are depriving our cells of optimal signaling and function.

Light exposure during the day is directly linked to improved HRV levels. Our eyes and skin prefer to receive signals from red, infra-red, and yellow wavelengths during sunrise and sunset, while they prefer blue, green, violet, and ultraviolet light during the middle of the day. Sun exposure will do this naturally, while our workplaces, cars, and homes will not—at least not yet. Circadian lighting technology is being developed by many companies at the time of this writing.

As sunlight is directly linked to HRV levels, it is highly recommended that you get outside and get direct sunlight on your skin each day. Doing this at several different times of day is

Activate your VAGUS NERVE

an even better option. The best times to get outside are within 30 minutes of sunrise, two or three times during the day, and within 30 minutes of sunset. Even better, spend the entire day outdoors whenever possible. You are far less likely to burn your skin during the day if your body senses the sunrise and is pre-conditioned to the UV light that we experience during the daytime.

Supplementation

Because our diets lack nutrient density and our environments have decreased our microbiome diversity, supplementation is a smart way to ensure our cells get the correct micronutrients and signals that will allow them to function optimally. Contrary to prior belief, supplements are not a waste of money, as long as they are taken by the right person for the right reason. Using functional lab testing, we can determine the best supplements for each individual to reach their optimal cellular function. There are, however, some basic nutrients and signaling supplements that can help all of us. Note that this is intended as general advice. You should speak to your primary health care practitioner prior to starting or stopping any medications or supplementation that has been prescribed or recommended to you.

Probiotics

Antibiotic use, C-sections, and diets of poor nutrient density have led us to have poor bacterial diversity and low levels of good bacteria in our gut. Testing to confirm which bacterial species are present is the optimal choice, but the majority of us will need to support our gut and skin microbiome using probiotics. Probiotics are bacteria that are produced externally.

When ingested, they can help improve bacterial diversity and growth of good bacterial colonies. These are different from prebiotics, which are generally derived from fiber and act as food for the bacteria to produce vitamins and minerals for us.

When choosing a probiotic, I recommend spore-based, naturally formed bacterial species, such as Bacillus, which are formed naturally in soil. These probiotics help to fill the voids that are left when other bacteria die off. Probiotics that must be refrigerated tend to have a very low absorption rate (5 to 10 percent) when compared with spore-based probiotics and those that don't need to be refrigerated. The question that I ask of probiotics that must be refrigerated is that if the bacteria can't withstand room temperature, how will they get past the acid of the stomach and live through our higher body temperature?

MegaSporeBiotic is my preferred probiotic option for most patients on a maintenance protocol. It has a very high absorption rate, does not need to be refrigerated, and contains Bacillus species that can help fill the voids left by many different types of missing bacterial species, not just Lactobacillus and Bifidobacteria, which are the main species covered by the majority of probiotics.

Omega-3 Fatty Acids

High-quality omega-3 fatty acids are not found in our Standard American Diets and diets of poor nutrient density. Often called fish oils, they are most commonly derived from fish, but can also come from certain plant sources, which are the preferred source for vegans.

The issue with most ingestible omega-3 oils is that they are artificially formed from the natural sources and this processing decreases the effectiveness of these sources. The natural form contains triglycerides while the processed form contains ethyl esters. Ethyl esters tend to taste and smell much fishier than triglycerides.

When choosing a high-quality source of omega-3 fatty acids, I highly recommend going for the triglyceride type, as it is natural and contains a high quantity of EPA and DHA, both of which are necessary for brain function and anti-inflammatory effects in the body. EPA and DHA improve nerve function, including VN function, as they are required for myelination of nerves and provide anti-inflammatory effects. Supplementation with omega-3 fatty acids has also been shown recently to improve heart rate variability in obese children. I personally use capsules from Ortho Molecular Products and Designs for Health, both for my patients as well as my family.

5-HTP for Serotonin

This section is specific to dealing with issues of low mood and depression. Sadly, depression and mental health issues are very common in North America today, and research shows that anti-depressant medications may actually be causing more of a problem. A long-term study published in 2014 by O'Regan et al. showed that patients with depression had a reduced HRV, and that these rates are actually made worse by anti-depressant medications that are trying to improve serotonin levels.

The precursor to serotonin is called 5-HTP. It can be used as an effective supplement to allow your body the opportunity to build its own serotonin. Most cases of depression are due to serotonin imbalance, and organic acid functional testing, which I use with nearly every patient that comes into my office, can actually tell our patients whether they have too much serotonin and use it up very quickly, or if they are running low on its production.

One thing to keep in mind is that the vast majority of serotonin production is aided by the gut microbiome. A balanced microbiome will produce a good amount of serotonin and allow mood to be balanced while an unbalanced microbiome will do the opposite, leading to a higher risk of mental health issues.

Coffee Enemas

In more severe cases of bowel motility issues, especially when people are chronically constipated and unable to void their bowels for quite some time, enemas can be highly effective. A strong coffee enema is a great and simple option with a very high efficacy level. In the book *Why Isn't My Brain Working?*, Dr. Datis Kharrazian discusses how the caffeine found in coffee strongly stimulates the nicotinic ACh receptors, the same receptors that the vagus affects through its release of acetylcholine. Caffeine stimulates these receptors in the gut, causing an artificial urge to void the bowels through a bowel movement.

To effectively use this tool to re-train vagus nerve, you must suppress that urge for as long as possible. By suppressing the urge to go, you are actually causing an axis in your brain to fire (the frontopontine vagal enteric axis), essentially forcing the vagus and brain to become highly active and learn to

Activate your VAGUS NERVE

reactivate these gut motility nerves. If you do this regularly over time, the vagus nerve will be retrained and will be able to release stools without needing the external support of a coffee enema.

If chronic constipation and poor liver detoxification are issues for you, then this process is an effective tool to help you clear out the bowels and get the toxins out of your body more efficiently. Doing this correctly and suppressing the urge to void for as long as possible, you will actually be training the VN to learn how to fire and affect the nerves that control gut motility.

CHAPTER 16

PASSIVE METHODS TO ACTIVATE THE VAGUS NERVE

In addition to all the active exercises that you can perform on your own, there are passive treatments that can have profound effects on the activation of the vagus nerve. Some of these involve using certain equipment or visiting a health care provider, while others you can do in the comfort of your own home. Remember to discuss these options with your primary health care provider prior to beginning any type of treatment.

Auricular Acupuncture

Acupuncture is an effective form of therapy for many conditions, and I have seen its spectacular effects firsthand using it with my patients as a hands-on chiropractor. If you recall, one of the four types of signals that vagus controls is sensation to specific parts of the external ear, or auricle: the entire con-cha, the crus of the helix, and the tragus. As such, stimulation of these specific regions will have effects that can stimulate the function of the vagus nerve. As we discussed in Chapter 3, the vagus nerve receives purely sensory information through its auricular branch via the central and anterior part of the ear. By using acupuncture, we can increase the flow of infor-mation in the auricular branch of VN, and thus increase VN activation.

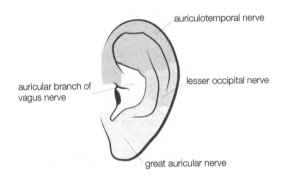

auriculotemporal nerve

lesser occipital nerve

auricular branch of
vagus nerve

great auricular nerve

A significant and growing body of research shows that acupuncture and transcutaneous vagus nerve stimulation through the auricular branch of the VN yields positive effects in many patients suffering from depression, anxiety, epilepsy, LPS-induced inflammation, tinnitus, and highly active pain receptors. The best part about this form of treatment is that it is effective without being invasive.

There is also a growing trend in the health care community centered around the activation of the vagus nerve through electrical stimulation. This is done by surgically implanting an electrical stimulation device on the vagus nerve itself. Acupuncture is significantly safer than and just as effective as this invasive technique. In fact, auricular acupuncture and implanted vagus nerve stimulation devices engage the exact same neural pathways. Given the choice, I would personally choose acupuncture every time.

Massage Therapy and Reflexology

Massage therapy is a great tool to help us relax. Immediately following a good massage, I personally move slower, breathe deeper, and see the world in a more positive light. Unless your therapist is hitting some severely tender spots, most people feel quite relaxed and refreshed following a massage. This feeling can be the epitome of parasympathetic activation and sympathetic deactivation.

Not surprisingly, many different techniques of massage have been linked to increases in HRV levels or improved vagal tone including Chinese head massage; traditional Thai shoulder, neck, and head massage; traditional back massage; and even self-massage.

For my many patients that have trouble getting relaxed, I also recommend trying reflexology. Ever since my mom learned to practice reflexology, I had been open to the possibilities and was the first to volunteer as a patient when she was learning. Every time she would work on my feet, I would fall asleep, even as a teenager. For this reason, I was not surprised when I found a research article showing that patients treated with foot reflexology showed significantly increased HRV levels and lower blood pressure levels 30 and 60 minutes after treatment.

Passive therapies like massage therapy and reflexology can have enormously beneficial effects on our health when they help us to relax and increase vagus nerve function. This is just another great reason to get regularly scheduled massages!

Visceral Manipulation

Visceral manipulation (VM) is a less common therapy but one that is very effective when practiced correctly. Typically practiced by osteopaths, chiropractors, naturopaths, and other health care providers, VM is the gentle physical manipulation of the organs of the abdomen, thus increasing blood flow to areas that are not functioning optimally. Patients can use this feedback tool on their own, if learned correctly.

As we know, the vagus nerve innervates all of the abdominal organs including the liver, gallbladder, pancreas, kidneys, spleen, stomach, small intestine, and ascending and transverse sections of the large intestine. For the VN to affect these organs and signal the brain about organ function, it is imperative that the organs function optimally. Physical restrictions can build up in these organs that can only be altered by physical manipulation and mobilization. Improving blood flow to these organs can have significant beneficial results on organ health and allow the VN to send signals relating to optimal function.

Visceral manipulation therapists use gently applied hands-on therapy to find areas of altered or decreased motion within the viscera and release restrictions within these visceral organs. The treatment involves a gentle compression, mobilization, or elongation of the soft tissues. Finding a certified visceral manipulation therapist in your area may be a good idea, especially for those people dealing with dysfunction with detoxification or with liver, gallbladder, or kidney pain.

Chiropractic Care

Mechanical neck and back pain are common around the world. They have become far more prevalent over the last 20 years as our jobs and careers have become significantly more sedentary and the majority of them require us to sit in front of a computer for hours on end. As a chiropractor, I have treated thousands of patients dealing with pain in their neck and back as a result of sitting in this position for many hours each day.

When joints are not moved through their full range for a long period of time, the muscles around them can become quite stiff and weak. As a result, the joints can become mildly misaligned and lead to pain. Mechanical joint pain caused by lack of motion is more common than pain from overuse of a joint. In my practice, I have found it to be absolutely true that if you don't use it, you lose it—function of a joint, that is.

A 2015 study in the *Journal of Chiropractic Medicine* showed that in patients with neck pain, spinal manipulation performed by a chiropractor led to significant positive changes in blood pressure and heart rate variability, significantly improving VN activity. A 2009 study published in the *Journal of Manipulative and Physiological Therapeutics* yielded similar positive results for patients with lower back pain. Both of these studies concluded that the reduction in pain levels allowed patients to breathe slower and improve their vagus nerve function, and that chiropractic manipulation provided a positive effect on patients' mechanical function. Especially when one is in pain, chiropractic care can be a very effective method of therapy and can have a significant benefit for VN and parasympathetic activity.

Activate your VAGUS NERVE

Electrical Stimulation

Over the past hundred or so years, researchers have conducted tests to learn about the effects of the vagus nerve. One technique involved stimulating the VN using electrical stimulation devices on experimental animals. In addition to learning about the importance of the VN itself, researchers eventually determined that by electrically stimulating the vagus nerve, they were able to supplement its functions.

In the 1980s and early 1990s, experiments were done to show that stimulation of the vagus in the neck was effective in reducing seizure activity in dogs. This research led to dedicated clinical trials that produced vagus nerve stimulation (VNS) devices that could be implanted in the neck. These devices were approved by the FDA in 1997 for the treatment of epilepsy, and in 2005 for the treatment of chronic, treatment-resistant depression. Since that time, researchers and corporations have been producing and improving devices to electrically stimulate the VN for various medical conditions including headaches, bipolar disorder, treatment-resistant anxiety disorders, Alzheimer's disease, and obesity. Today, the most common clinically used electrical VNS device is the NCP System from Cyberonics, which is implanted on the left vagus nerve during an outpatient procedure. This unit is used to treat patients dealing with severe treatment-resistant depression and/or epilepsy.

Right-side VNS is effective in animal models of epilepsy and seizures, but is not known to have strong effects on depressive symptoms. Preliminary human trials are promising and have yielded positive effects, and some companies have already begun creating vagus nerve stimulation tools that can be used for various conditions. The CardioFit system from BioControl Medical uses right-side VNS to activate efferent fibers and aid in treatment of heart failure, while the FitNeSS System from BioControl Medical is designed to activate afferent fibers, thus helping to reduce side effects of electrical vagal stimulation.

Typical surgical risks associated with this procedure include infection, pain, scarring, difficulty swallowing, and vocal cord paralysis. Side effects from implanted electrical stimulation devices include voice changes, hoarseness, throat pain, cough, headache, chest pain, breathing problems (especially during exercise), difficulty swallowing, abdominal pain, nausea, tingling of the skin, insomnia, and bradycardia (slowing of the heart rate). Although many of these are temporary, they can be severe and can last permanently.

There are other devices for electrical stimulation that do not need to be implanted, though they show mixed results and are approved for certain conditions only at this point. The NEMOS system from Cerbomed is a transcutaneous VNS device that is applied to the part of the ear that is innervated by vagus. It has been cleared for treatment of epilepsy and depression in Europe at this time. The gammaCore device from US-based company electroCore has been granted clearance in Europe for acute treatment of cluster headaches, migraines, and medication overuse headaches. The gammaCore is a handheld portable device with two flat stimulation contact surfaces that are applied to the side of the neck over the vagus nerve. Larger trials are underway for treatment of other conditions.

As promising as electrical stimulation of the vagus nerve is, I would recommend using daily exercises and forming beneficial habits before trying external equipment such as electrical stimulation devices. If you are able to produce a strong effect

Activate your VAGUS NERVE

on your vagus nerve activity using the exercises discussed previously, I feel the symptoms will improve drastically without unnecessary risks and costs.

Actively using the active exercises described in Chapter 15 and the passive treatment methods described in this chapter can help you improve symptoms of anxiety, depression, epilepsy, chronic inflammatory conditions, autoimmune conditions, and cardiovascular conditions. As we well know, the body has a strong anti-inflammatory system, and if the VN is exercised and functioning correctly, this system can improve overall health significantly by keeping inflammation levels in check.

CONCLUSION

A candle loses nothing by lighting another candle.
  —Father James Keller

I am grateful that you have taken the time to read my work. I truly hope that it has inspired and educated you to take back control of your health.

Now that you comprehend the nature of the parasympathetic nervous system and the extent to which the VN transmits information, the power is in your hands to improve its function and take back your health. For some of you, these strategies and protocols will have profound effects that drastically improve your energy, digestion, inflammation, and pain, while for others, this may simply be the first step in your journey.

Wherever you are in your health journey, take a moment to commit to becoming responsible for this knowledge. Share it with those around you—family, friends, and loved ones—who need to hear that there are answers for what may be ailing them.

For those of you who make significant improvement with some of the simple changes outlined in this book, keep up the good work and form healthier habits. For those that need someone to hold your hand through the journey, that is good and nothing to feel ashamed of at all. Seek out forward-thinking health care practitioners that do not practice in-the-box medicine. Find someone to help you along your journey, who will actually care about you as an individual and guide you to determine the root cause of your issues.

You can connect with me through my website or by using the social media links listed below. Feel free reach out to me personally if you feel that you need some support to determine your next steps to improved overall health. I am truly grateful for each and every one of you, and I wish you the best on your journey.

APPENDIX

Daily Practices
for Activating the Vagus Nerve

Gargling *2x daily*	Keep a cup beside your bathroom sink. Use it to gargle twice each day, when you brush your teeth in the morning and at night.
Gag reflex activation *2x daily*	When you brush your teeth in the morning and at night, use your toothbrush to stimulate the gag reflex on both the left and right side of your soft palate.
Humming *2x daily*	During your daily commute or to bookend your day, practice humming deep in your throat. You can use the word "om" and hold the vibration in your throat for as long as you can exhale.
Cold shower *1x daily*	End your daily shower with one minute of cold water (as cold as possible) and practice breathing through the shock of the temperature change. As this becomes easier, increase the time by 30 to 60 seconds every three days until your entire shower is taken under cold water.
Deep breathing *3x daily*	Practice three to five minutes of deep breathing in a quiet space before each meal. This will help to calm you down and improve your digestion for each meal.
Sunlight exposure *3x daily*	Go outside and expose your skin to the sun within 30 minutes of sunrise, in the middle of the day, and within 30 minutes of the sunset, each time for a minimum of five minutes. If you live in a colder climate, expose your eyes to the light at each of these times for two to three minutes, and practice breathing through the cold each time you do.
Sleep on your side *Each night*	Put a pillow between your knees to keep you sleeping on your side each night.

Weekly Practices
for Activating the Vagus Nerve

Yoga/Pilates or light exercise *2–3x weekly*	Ensure you are moving your body and exercising at least twice per week. Create a routine that is non-negotiable, forcing you to create a habit of movement. Yoga, Pilates, and light exercise are great ways to get your body moving, practice optimal breathing patterns, and sweat out some toxins on a regular basis.
Social interaction *1–2x weekly*	Make a point of meeting with friends or family in person at least once each week. During these meetings, if the situation calls for it, laugh out loud, as much as you can! If you have trouble meeting with friends, join a weekly meeting group on Meetup or through a platform that is exciting to you.
Listening to music *2x weekly*	Make a point of relaxing to your favorite music at home a couple of times per week. Doing this in the car while driving is not optimal as you are under the stress of driving, so take time to close your eyes and listen to something soothing like Mozart's "K.448 Two Pianos" at least twice per week.
Green/Clean/Lean grocery shopping *1–2x weekly*	Don't buy foods that shouldn't be in your house. Keep your pantry clean and it will be easier to keep your body clean and functioning with good nutrients.
Meditation and mindfulness practice *3–7x weekly*	If you are just beginning to practice meditation or mindfulness practice, take five to ten minutes 3x each week to focus on your breath and close your eyes. As this becomes easier, increase the time period as well as the frequency. Some of the most productive people on the planet practice meditation for up to one hour each day, and the strongest even wake up to practice very early each morning.

Activate your VAGUS NERVE

Monthly Practices
for Activating the Vagus Nerve

Check your supplements *1x monthly*	Take a good-quality probiotic, omega-3, and multivitamin that should be refilled once per month. For a more personalized protocol, visit a functional medicine practitioner to have functional lab testing done and interpreted by an experienced professional that knows how to eliminate root causes and get you off the supplements in a timely manner.
Massage therapy, chiropractic care, or visceral manipulation *2x monthly*	Have a combination of massage, reflexology, chiropractic care, or visceral manipulation done twice each month. This will keep your body in alignment, and keep your organs and muscles functioning optimally. Find a provider or clinic that you trust and stick with them—they will get to know your body and the common issues that may afflict you. The best providers will refer you out when they find something that needs further evaluation.
Acupuncture treatment *1–2x monthly*	Due to the high efficacy of acupuncture, I recommend having treatment done at least once each month to send signals via your vagus nerve and keep it functioning optimally. Find a reliable, experienced, and clean acupuncture practitioner near you that you trust and who is aware of strategies to help activate the vagus nerve through points in the ear.

BIBLIOGRAPHY

Anderson, Scott C., John F. Cryan, and Ted Dinan. *The Psychobiotic Revolution*. Washington, D.C.: National Geographic, 2017.

Assenza, Giovanni, Chiara Campana, Gabriella Colicchio, et al. "Transcutaneous and Invasive Vagal Nerve Stimulations Engage the Same Neural Pathways: In-vivo Human Evidence." *Brain Stimulation* 10, no. 4 (2017): 853–54. doi: 10.1016/j.brs.2017.03.005.

Austin, Evan, Amy Huang, Tony Adar, et al. "Electronic Device Generated Light Increases Reactive Oxygen Species in Human Fibroblasts." *Lasers in Surgery and Medicine* 50, no. 6 (2018): 689–95. doi: 10.1002/lsm.22794.

Azam, Muhammad Abid, Joel Katz, Samantha R. Fashler, et al. "Heart Rate Variability Is Enhanced in Controls but Not Maladaptive Perfectionists during Brief Mindfulness Meditation following Stress-Induction: A Stratified-Randomized Trial." *International Journal of Psychophysiology* 98, no. 1 (2015): 27–34. doi: 10.1016/j.ijpsycho.2015.06.005.

Baharav, A., S. Kotagal, V. Gibbons, et al. "Fluctuations in Autonomic Nervous Activity during Sleep Displayed by Power Spectrum Analysis of Heart Rate Variability." *Neurology* 45, no. 6 (1995): 1183–187. doi: 10.1212/wnl.45.6.1183.

Balzarotti, S., F. Biassoni, B. Colombo, et al. "Cardiac Vagal Control as a Marker of Emotion Regulation in Healthy Adults: A Review." *Biological Psychology* 130 (2017): 54–66. doi: 10.1016/j.biopsycho.2017.10.008.

Activate your VAGUS NERVE

Baumann, Christoph, Ulla Rakowski, and Reiner Buchhorn. "Omega-3 Fatty Acid Supplementation Improves Heart Rate Variability in Obese Children." *International Journal of Pediatrics* 2018 (2018): 1–5. doi: 10.1155/2018/8789604.

Bercik, P., A. J. Park, D. Sinclair, et al. "The Anxiolytic Effect of Bifidobacterium Longum NCC3001 Involves Vagal Pathways for Gut-Brain Communication." *Neurogastroenterology and Motility* 23, no. 12 (2011): 1132–39. doi: 10.1111/j.1365-2982.2011.01796.x.

Bonaz, Bruno, Thomas Bazin, and Sonia Pellissier. "The Vagus Nerve at the Interface of the Microbiota-Gut-Brain Axis." *Frontiers in Neuroscience* 12 (2018): 49. doi: 10.3389/fnins.2018.00049.

Bravo, Javier A., Paul Forsythe, Marianne V. Chew, et al. "Ingestion of Lactobacillus Strain Regulates Emotional Behavior and Central GABA Receptor Expression in a Mouse via the Vagus Nerve." *Proceedings of the National Academy of Sciences* 108, no. 38 (2011): 16050–55. doi: 10.1073/pnas.1102999108.

Buettner, Dan. *The Blue Zones.* Washington, DC: National Geographic, 2008.

Cacho, Nicole, and Josef Neu. "Manipulation of the Intestinal Microbiome in Newborn Infants." *Advances in Nutrition* 5, no. 1 (2014): 114–18. doi: 10.3945/an.113.004820.

Canterini, Claire-Charlotte, Isabelle Gaubil-Kaladjian, Séverine Vatin, et al. "Rapid Eating Is Linked to Emotional Eating in Obese Women Relieving from Bariatric Surgery." *Obesity Surgery* 28, no. 2 (2018): 526–31. doi: 10.1007/s11695-017-2890-4.

Chapleau, Mark W., and Rasna Sabharwal. "Methods of Assessing Vagus Nerve Activity and Reflexes." *Heart Failure Reviews* 16, no. 2 (2011): 109–27. doi: 10.1007/s10741-010-9174-6.

Chuang, Chih-Yuan, Wei-Ru Han, Pei-Chun Li, et al. "Effects of Music Therapy on Subjective Sensations and Heart Rate Variability in Treated Cancer Survivors: A Pilot Study." *Complementary Therapies in Medicine* 18, no. 5 (2010): 224–26. doi: 10.1016/j.ctim.2010.08.003.

Cole, Christopher R., Eugene H. Blackstone, Fredric J. Pashkow, et al. "Heart-Rate Recovery Immediately after Exercise as a Predictor of Mortality." *New England Journal of Medicine* 341, no. 18 (1999): 1351–57. doi: 10.1056/nejm199910283411804.

Córdova, Ezequiel, Elena Maiolo, Marcelo Corti, et al. "Neurological Manifestations of Chagas' Disease." *Neurological Research* 32, no. 3 (2010): 238–44. doi: 10.1179/016164110x12644252260637.

Costes, Léa, Guy Boeckxstaens, Wouter J de Jonge, et al. "Neural Networks in Intestinal Immunoregulation." *Organogenesis* 9, no. 3 (07, 2013): 216–23. doi: 10.4161/org.25646.

Cryan, John F., and Timothy G. Dinan. "Mind-Altering Microorganisms: The Impact of the Gut Microbiota on Brain and Behaviour." *Nature Reviews Neuroscience* 13, no. 10 (2012): 701–12. doi: 10.1038/nrn3346.

Dang, Xitong, Brian P. Eliceiri, Andrew Baird, et al. "CHRFAM7A: A Human-Specific α7-Nicotinic Acetylcholine Receptor Gene Shows Differential Responsiveness of Human Intestinal Epithelial Cells to LPS." *The FASEB Journal* 29, no. 6 (2015): 2292–302. doi: 10.1096/fj.14-268037.

de Jonge, Wouter J. "The Gut's Little Brain in Control of Intestinal Immunity." *ISRN Gastroenterology* 2013 (2013): 1–17. doi: 10.1155/2013/630159.

de Lartigue, Guillaume, and Charlene Diepenbroek. "Novel Developments in Vagal Afferent Nutrient Sensing and Its Role in Energy Homeostasis." *Current Opinion in Pharmacology* 31 (2016): 38–43. doi: 10.1016/j.coph.2016.08.007.

de Lartigue, Guillaume. "Role of the Vagus Nerve in the Development and Treatment of Diet-Induced Obesity." *The Journal of Physiology* 594, no. 20 (2016): 5791–815. doi: 10.1113/jp271538.

de Lartigue, Guillaume, Claire Barbier de La Serre, and Helen E. Raybould. "Vagal Afferent Neurons in High Fat Diet-Induced Obesity; Intestinal Microflora, Gut Inflammation and Cholecystokinin." *Physiology & Behavior* 105, no. 1 (2011): 100–05. doi: 10.1016/j.physbeh.2011.02.040.

Dinan, Timothy G., and John F. Cryan. "Gut Instincts: Microbiota as a Key Regulator of Brain Development, Ageing, and Neurodegeneration." *The Journal of Physiology* 595, no. 2 (2017): 489–503. doi: 10.1113/jp273106.

Dipatrizio, Nicholas V. "Endocannabinoids in the Gut." *Cannabis and Cannabinoid Research* 1, no. 1 (2016): 67–77. doi: 10.1089/can.2016.0001.

"Discover Visceral Manipulation." The Barral Institute. http://www.discovervm.com.

Forsythe, Paul, John Bienenstock, and Wolfgang A. Kunze. "Vagal Pathways for Microbiome-Brain-Gut Axis Communication." *Advances in Experimental Medicine and Biology* 817 (2014), 115–33. doi: 10.1007/978-1-4939-0897-4_5.

Goehler, Lisa E., Su Mi Park, Noel Opitz, et al. "Campylobacter Jejuni Infection Increases Anxiety-like Behavior in the Holeboard: Possible Anatomical Substrates for Viscerosensory Modulation of Exploratory Behavior." *Brain, Behavior, and Immunity* 22, no. 3 (2008): 354–66. doi: 10.1016/j.bbi.2007.08.009.

Grippo, Angela J., Damon G. Lamb, C. Sue Carter, et al. "Social Isolation Disrupts Autonomic Regulation of the Heart and Influences Negative Affective Behaviors." *Biological Psychiatry* 62, no. 10 (2007): 1162–70. doi: 10.1016/j.biopsych.2007.04.011.

Activate your VAGUS NERVE

Hajiasgharzadeh, Khalil, and Behzad Baradaran. "Cholinergic Anti-Inflammatory Pathway and the Liver." *Advanced Pharmaceutical Bulletin* 7, no. 4 (12, 2017): 507–13. doi: 10.15171/apb.2017.063.

Halliez, Marie C. M., and André G. Buret. "Gastrointestinal Parasites and the Neural Control of Gut Functions." *Frontiers in Cellular Neuroscience* 25, no. 9 (2015): 425. doi: 10.3389/fncel.2015.00452.

Halliez, Marie C. M., Jean-Paul Motta, Troy D. Feener, et al. "Giardia Duodenalis Induces Paracellular Bacterial Translocation and Causes Postinfectious Visceral Hypersensitivity." *American Journal of Physiology-Gastrointestinal and Liver Physiology* 310, no. 8 (2016): G574–85. doi: 10.1152/ajpgi.00144.2015.

Henriquez, Victor M., Geralyn M. Schulz, Steven Bielamowicz, et al. "Laryngeal Reflex Responses Are Not Modulated during Human Voice and Respiratory Tasks." *The Journal of Physiology* 585, pt. 3 (2007): 779–89. doi: 10.1113/jphysiol.2007.143438.

Howland, Robert H. "Vagus Nerve Stimulation." *Current Behavioral Neuroscience Reports* 1, no. 2 (2014) 64–73. doi: 10.1007/s40473-014-0010-5.

Jardine, David L., Wouter Wieling, Michele Brignole, et al. "The Pathophysiology of the Vasovagal Response." *Heart Rhythm* 15, no. 6 (2018): 921–29. doi: 10.1016/j.hrthm.2017.12.013.

Kaczmarczyk, R., D. Tejera, B. J. Simon, et al. "Microglia Modulation through External Vagus Nerve Stimulation in a Murine Model of Alzheimer's Disease." *Journal of Neurochemistry* (2017). doi: 10.1111/jnc.14284.

Kelly, John R., Chiara Minuto, John F. Cryan, et al. "Cross Talk: The Microbiota and Neurodevelopmental Disorders." *Frontiers in Neuroscience* 11 (2017). doi: 10.3389/fnins.2017.00490.

Kentish, Stephen J., Claudine L. Frisby, David J. Kennaway, et al. "Circadian Variation in Gastric Vagal Afferent Mechanosensitivity." *Journal of Neuroscience* 33, no. 49 (2013): 19238–42. doi: 10.1523/jneurosci.3846-13.2013.

Kharrazian, Datis. *Why Isn't My Brain Working?: A Revolutionary Understanding of Brain Decline and Effective Strategies to Recover Your Brain's Health.* Carlsbad, CA: Elephant Press, 2013.

Kok, Bethany E., and Barbara L. Fredrickson. "Upward Spirals of the Heart: Autonomic Flexibility, as Indexed by Vagal Tone, Reciprocally and Prospectively Predicts Positive Emotions and Social Connectedness." *Biological Psychology* 85, no. 3 (12, 2010): 432–36. doi: 10.1016/j.biopsycho.2010.09.005.

Krygier, Jonathan R., James A. J. Heathers, Sara Shahrestani, et al. "Mindfulness Meditation, Well-Being, and Heart Rate Variability: A Preliminary Investigation into the Impact of Intensive Vipassana Meditation." *International Journal of Psychophysiology* 89, no. 3 (09, 2013): 305–13. doi: 10.1016/j.ijpsycho.2013.06.017.

Lin, Guiping, Qiuling Xiang, Xiaodong Fu, et al. "Heart Rate Variability Biofeedback Decreases Blood Pressure in Prehypertensive Subjects by Improving Autonomic Function and Baroreflex." *The Journal of Alternative and Complementary Medicine* 18, no. 2 (2012): 143–52. doi: 10.1089/acm.2010.0607.

Lin, Lung-Chang, Mei-Wen Lee, Ruey-Chang Wei, et al. "Mozart K.448 Listening Decreased Seizure Recurrence and Epileptiform Discharges in Children with First Unprovoked Seizures: A Randomized Controlled Study." *BMC Complementary and Alternative Medicine* 14, no. 17 (2014). doi: 10.1186/1472-6882-14-17.

Lipton, Bruce H. *The Biology of Belief: Unleashing the Power of Consciousness, Matter, and Miracles.* Carlsbad, CA: Hay House, Inc., 2005.

Lu, Wan-An., Gua-Yang Chen, Cheng-Deng Kuo. "Foot Reflexology Can Increase Vagal Modulation, Decrease Sympathetic Modulation, and Lower Blood Pressure in Healthy Subjects and Patients with Coronary Artery Disease." *Alternative Therapies in Health and Medicine* 17, no. 4 (2011): 8–14. https://www.ncbi.nlm.nih.gov/pubmed/22314629.

Luyer, Misha D., Jan Willem M. Greve, M'hamed Hadfoune, et al. "Nutritional Stimulation of Cholecystokinin Receptors Inhibits Inflammation via the Vagus Nerve." *The Journal of Experimental Medicine* 202, no. 8 (2005): 1023–29. doi: 10.1084/jem.20042397.

Mager, Donald E., Ruiqian Wan, Martin Brown, et al. "Caloric Restriction and Intermittent Fasting Alter Spectral Measures of Heart Rate and Blood Pressure Variability in Rats." *The FASEB Journal* 20, no. 6 (2006): 631–37. doi: 10.1096/fj.05-5263com.

Mäkinen, Tiina M., Matti Mäntysaari, Tiina Pääkkönen, et al. "Autonomic Nervous Function During Whole-Body Cold Exposure Before and After Cold Acclimation." *Aviation, Space, and Environmental Medicine* 79, no. 9 (09, 2008): 875–82. doi: 10.3357/asem.2235.2008.

Mattsson, Mats-Olof, Olga Zeni, Myrtill Simkó, et al. "Editorial: Effects of Combined EMF Exposures and Co-exposures." *Frontiers in Public Health* 6, no. 230 (2018). doi: 10.3389/fpubh.2018.00230.

Mayo Clinic Staff. "Vagus Nerve Stimulation." Mayo Clinic. March 21, 2018. https://www.mayoclinic.org/tests-procedures/vagus-nerve-stimulation/about/pac-20384565.

Mercante, Beniamina, Franca Deriu, and Claire-Marie Rangon. "Auricular Neuromodulation: The Emerging Concept beyond the Stimulation of Vagus and Trigeminal Nerves." Medicines 5, no. 1 (2018): 10. doi: 10.3390/medicines5010010.

Morris III, George L., David Gloss, Jeffrey Buchhalter, et al. "Evidence-Based Guideline Update: Vagus Nerve Stimulation for the Treatment of Epilepsy." *Epilepsy Currents* 13, no. 6 (2013): 297–303. doi: 10.5698/1535-7597-13.6.297.

Mukai, K. and S. J. Galli. "Basophils." *Encyclopedia of Life Sciences* (6, 2013). doi: 10.1002/9780470015902.a0001120.pub3.

Müller, Mattea, Emanuel Canfora, and Ellen Blaak. "Gastrointestinal Transit Time, Glucose Homeostasis and Metabolic Health: Modulation by Dietary Fibers." *Nutrients* 10, no. 3 (2018): 275. doi: 10.3390/nu10030275.

Myers, William. "How Mouth Breathing Impacts Dental Health." Dr. William Myers: Cosmetic, General, Implant Dentistry. November 04, 2014. https://www.drwilliammyers.com/mouth-breathing-impacts-dental-health/.

National Sleep Foundation. "Understanding Sleep Cycles." Sleep.org. Accessed December 13, 2018. https://sleep.org/articles/what-happens-during-sleep/.

Opazo, Maria C., Elizabeth M. Ortega-Rocha, Irenice Coronado-Arrázola, et al. "Intestinal Microbiota Influences Non-Intestinal Related Autoimmune Diseases." *Frontiers in Microbiology* 12, no. 9 (2018). doi: 10.3389/fmicb.2018.00432.

O'Regan, C., R. A. Kenny, H. Cronin, et al. "Antidepressants Strongly Influence the Relationship between Depression and Heart Rate Variability: Findings from The Irish Longitudinal Study on Ageing (TILDA)." *Psychological Medicine* 45, no. 03 (2015): 623–36. doi: 10.1017/s0033291714001767.

O'Toole, Paul W., and Ian B. Jeffery. "Gut Microbiota and Aging." *Science* 350, no. 6265 (2015): 1214–15. doi:10.1126/science.aac8469.

Owyang, Chung, and Andrea Heldsinger. "Vagal Control of Satiety and Hormonal Regulation of Appetite." *Journal of Neurogastroenterology and Motility* 17, no. 4 (2011): 338–48. doi: 10.5056/jnm.2011.17.4.338.

Pelot, Nicole A., and Warren M. Grill. "Effects of Vagal Neuromodulation on Feeding Behavior." *Brain Research* 15, no. 1693 pt. B (2018): 180–87. doi: 10.1016/j.brainres.2018.02.003.

Polyzoidis, Stavros, Triantafyllia Koletsa, Smaro Panagiotidou, et al. "Mast Cells in Meningiomas and Brain Inflammation." *Journal of Neuro-inflammation* 12, no. 1 (2015): 170. doi: 10.1186/s12974-015-0388-3.

Pramanik, Tapas, Hari Om Sharma, Suchita Mishra, et al. "Immediate Effect of Slow Pace Bhastrika Pranayama on Blood Pressure and Heart Rate." *The Journal of Alternative and Complementary Medicine* 15, no. 3 (2009): 293–95. doi: 10.1089/acm.2008.0440.

Rechlin, Thomas, Maria Weis, Kurt Schneider, et al. "Does Bright-light Therapy Influence Autonomic Heart-rate Parameters?" *Journal of Affective Disorders* 34, no. 2 (1995): 131–37. doi: 10.1016/0165-0327(95)00010-k.

Roager, Henrik M., Lea B. S. Hansen, Martin I. Bahl, et al. "Colonic Transit Time Is Related to Bacterial Metabolism and Mucosal Turnover in the Gut." *Nature Microbiology* 1, no. 9 (2016). doi: 10.1038/nmicrobiol.2016.93.

Rosas-Ballina, Mauricio, and Kevin J. Tracey. "The Neurology of the Immune System: Neural Reflexes Regulate Immunity." *Neuron* 64, no. 1 (2009): 28–32. doi: 10.1016/j.neuron.2009.09.039.

Roy, Richard A., Jean P. Boucher, and Alain S. Comtois. "Heart Rate Variability Modulation After Manipulation in Pain-Free Patients vs. Patients in Pain." *Journal of Manipulative and Physiological Therapeutics* 32, no. 4 (2009): 277–86. doi: 10.1016/j.jmpt.2009.03.003.

Sachis, Paul, Dawna Armstrong, Laurence Becker, et al. "Myelination of the Human Vagus Nerve from 24 Weeks Postconceptional Age to Adolescence." *Journal of Neuropathology and Experimental Neurology* 41, no. 4 (7, 1982). doi: 10.1097/00005072-198207000-00009.

Samsel, Anthony, and Stephanie Seneff. "Glyphosate Pathways to Modern Diseases VI: Prions, Amyloidoses and Autoimmune Neurological Diseases." *Journal of Biological Physics and Chemistry* 17, no. 1 (2017). doi: 10.4024/25sa16a.jbpc.17.01.

Sandhu, Kiran V., Eoin Sherwin, Harriët Schellekens, et al. "Feeding the Microbiota-Gut-Brain Axis: Diet, Microbiome, and Neuropsychiatry." *Translational Research* 179 (2017): 223–44. doi: 10.1016/j.trsl.2016.10.002.

Schweighöfer, Hanna, Christoph Rummel, Joachim Roth, et al. "Modulatory Effects of Vagal Stimulation on Neurophysiological Parameters and the Cellular Immune Response in the Rat Brain during Systemic Inflammation." *Intensive Care Medicine Experimental* 4, no. 1 (2016): 19. doi: 10.1186/s40635-016-0091-4.

Schwerdtfeger, Andreas, and Peter Friedrich-Mai. "Social Interaction Moderates the Relationship between Depressive Mood and Heart Rate Variability: Evidence from an Ambulatory Monitoring Study." *Health Psychology* 28, no. 4 (2009): 501–09. doi: 10.1037/a0014664.

Seneff, Stephanie, and Anthony Samsel. "Glyphosate, Pathways to Modern
    Diseases III: Manganese, Neurological Diseases, and Associated
    Pathologies." *Surgical Neurology International* 6, no. 1 (2015): 45. doi:
    10.4103/2152-7806.153876.

Shaffer, Fred, and J. P. Ginsberg. "An Overview of Heart Rate Variability
    Metrics and Norms." *Frontiers in Public Health* 28, no. 5 (2017): 258.
    doi: 10.3389/fpubh.2017.00258.

Sharashova, Ekaterina, Tom Wilsgaard, Ellisiv B. Mathiesen, et al. "Resting
    Heart Rate Predicts Incident Myocardial Infarction, Atrial Fibrillation,
    Ischaemic Stroke, and Death in the General Population: The Tromsø
    Study." *Journal of Epidemiology and Community Health* 70, no. 9 (2016):
    902–09. doi: 10.1136/jech-2015-206663.

Sherwin, Eoin, Kieran Rea, Timothy G. Dinan, et al. "A Gut (Microbiome)
    Feeling about the Brain." *Current Opinion in Gastroenterology* 32, no. 2
    (2016): 96–102. doi: 10.1097/mog.0000000000000244.

Spitoni, Grazia Fernanda, Cristina Ottaviani, Anna Maria Petta, et al.
    "Obesity Is Associated with Lack of Inhibitory Control and Impaired
    Heart Rate Variability Reactivity and Recovery in Response to Food
    Stimuli." *International Journal of Psychophysiology* 116 (2017): 77–84.
    doi: 10.1016/j.ijpsycho.2017.04.001.

Stecher, Bärbel. "The Roles of Inflammation, Nutrient Availability, and the
    Commensal Microbiota in Enteric Pathogen Infection." *Microbiology
    Specrum* 3, no. 3 (2015): 297–320. doi: 10.1128/microbiolspec.mbp
    -0008-2014.

Tan, Jason Por How, Jessica Elise Beilharz, Uté Vollmer-Conna, et al. "Heart
    Rate Variability as a Marker of Healthy Ageing." *International Journal of
    Cardiology* (2019). doi: 10.1016/j.ijcard.2018.08.005.

Thomson Healthcare Staff. *Physicians' Desk Reference*. Montvale, NJ:
    Physician's Desk Reference, 2008.

Tobaldini, Eleonora, Lino Nobili, Silvia Strada, et al. "Heart Rate Variability
    in Normal and Pathological Sleep." *Frontiers in Physiology* 4 (2013): 294.
    doi: 10.3389/fphys.2013.00294.

Tverdal, Aage, Vidar Hjellvik, and Randi Selmer. "Heart Rate and Mortality
    from Cardiovascular Causes: A 12 Year Follow-up Study of 379,843 Men
    and Women Aged 40–45 Years." *European Heart Journal* 29, no. 22 (2008):
    2772–81. doi: 10.1093/eurheartj/ehn435.

Uhm, Tae Gi, Byung Soo Kim, and Il Yup Chung. "Eosinophil Development,
    Regulation of Eosinophil-Specific Genes, and Role of Eosinophils in the
    Pathogenesis of Asthma." *Allergy, Asthma and Immunology Research* 4,
    no. 2 (2012): 68–79. doi: 10.4168/aair.2012.4.2.68.

"Underlying Causes of Dysautonomia." Dysautonomia International. http://www.dysautonomiainternational.org/page.php?ID=150.

VanElzakker, Michael B. "Chronic Fatigue Syndrome from Vagus Nerve Infection: A Psychoneuroimmunological Hypothesis." *Medical Hypotheses* 81, no. 3 (2013): 414–23. doi: 10.1016/j.mehy.2013.05.034.

Vivier, Eric, David H. Raulet, Alessandro Moretta, et al. "Innate or Adaptive Immunity? The Example of Natural Killer Cells." *Science* 331, no. 6013 (2011): 44–49. doi: 10.1126/science.1198687.

Wekerle, Hartmut. "The Gut–brain Connection: Triggering of Brain Autoimmune Disease by Commensal Gut Bacteria." *Rheumatology* 55, suppl. 2 (2016): ii68–ii75. doi: 10.1093/rheumatology/kew353.

White, James S. *Neuroscience.* 2nd ed. New York: McGraw-Hill Medical, 2008.

Win, Ni Ni, Anna Maria S. Jorgensen, Yu Sui Chen, et al. "Effects of Upper and Lower Cervical Spinal Manipulative Therapy on Blood Pressure and Heart Rate Variability in Volunteers and Patients with Neck Pain: A Randomized Controlled, Cross-Over, Preliminary Study." *Journal of Chiropractic Medicine* 14, no. 1 (2015): 1–9. doi: 10.1016/j.jcm.2014.12.005.

Wouters, Mira M., Maria Vicario, and Javier Santos. "The Role of Mast Cells in Functional GI Disorders." *Gut* 65, no. 1 (07, 2015): 155–68. doi: 10.1136/gutjnl-2015-309151.

Yamamoto, Takeshi, Toshihisa Kodama, Jaemin Lee, et al. "Anti-Allergic Role of Cholinergic Neuronal Pathway via α7 Nicotinic ACh Receptors on Mucosal Mast Cells in a Murine Food Allergy Model." *PLoS ONE* 9, no. 1 (2014): e85888. doi: 10.1371/journal.pone.0085888.

Yang, Cheryl C., Chi-Wan Lai, Hsien Yong Lai, et al. "Relationship between Electroencephalogram Slow-Wave Magnitude and Heart Rate Variability during Sleep in Humans." *Neuroscience Letters* 329, no. 2 (2002): 213–16. doi: 10.1016/s0304-3940(02)00661-4.

Yang, Jen-Lin, Gau-Yang Chen, and Cheng-Deng Kuo. "Comparison of Effect of 5 Recumbent Positions on Autonomic Nervous Modulation in Patients with Coronary Artery Disease." *Circulation Journal* 72, no. 6 (2008): 902–08. doi: 10.1253/circj.72.902.

Yim, Jongeun. "Therapeutic Benefits of Laughter in Mental Health: A Theoretical Review." *The Tohoku Journal of Experimental Medicine* 239, no. 3 (2016): 243–49. doi: 10.1620/tjem.239.243.

Young, Hayley A., and David Benton. "Heart-rate Variability: A Biomarker to Study the Influence of Nutrition on Physiological and Psychological Health?" Special issue *Behavioural Pharmacology* 29, no. 2 and 3 (2018): 140–51. doi: 10.1097/fbp.0000000000000383.

Yuan, Hsiangkuo, and Stephen D. Silberstein. "Vagus Nerve and Vagus Nerve Stimulation, a Comprehensive Review: Part II." *Headache: The Journal of Head and Face Pain* 56, no. 2 (2015): 259–66. doi: 10.1111/head.12650.

Yuen, Alan W., and J. W. Sander. "Can Natural Ways to Stimulate the Vagus Nerve Improve Seizure Control?" *Epilepsy & Behavior* 67 (2017): 105–10. doi: 10.1016/j.yebeh.2016.10.039.

Zabara, Jacob. "Inhibition of Experimental Seizures in Canines by Repetitive Vagal Stimulation." *Epilepsia* 33, no. 6 (1992): 1005–12. doi: 10.1111/j.1528-1157.1992.tb01751.x.

Zdrojewicz, Zygmunt, Ewelina Pachura, and Paulina Pachura. "The Thymus: A Forgotten, But Very Important Organ." *Advances in Clinical and Experimental Medicine* 25, no. 2 (2016): 369–75. doi: 10.17219/acem/58802.

Zinöcker, Marit, and Inge Lindseth. "The Western Diet–Microbiome-Host Interaction and Its Role in Metabolic Disease." *Nutrients* 10, no. 3 (2018): 365. doi: 10.3390/nu10030365.

Zoli, Michele, Susanna Pucci, Antonietta Vilella, et al. "Neuronal and Extraneuronal Nicotinic Acetylcholine Receptors." *Current Neuropharmacology* 16, no. 4 (05, 2018): 338–49. doi: 10.2174/1570159x15666170912110450.

INDEX

Activate your VAGUS NERVE

Cholecystokinin (CCK; gut hormone), 41–42, 82
Cholesterol, 43
Choline, 59, 60, 154
Cholinergic anti-inflammatory pathway, 24, 48, 52
Chronic fatigue syndrome, 91
Chronic obstructive pulmonary disease (COPD), 31
Chronic stress, 108–15
Chyme, 24
Circadian rhythm, 116–18
Coffee enemas, 160–61
Cold exposure, 140–42; and stress, 141
Colon, 78; ascending and transverse, 44; descending and sigmoid, 26
Computers. *See* Laptops
Constipation, 44, 76, 160–61
COPD (chronic obstructive pulmonary disease), 31
Cortisol, 38, 111
Coughing, 29, 30
Cravings, food, 54–55
Cryan, John, quoted, 54–55
Cryotherapy, 141, 142
Cyberonics NCP System, 167
Cytokines, 51

Deep cardiac plexus, 18
Depression, 120, 159–60
Diabesity, defined, 37
Diabetes, 37–38, 41, 42
Diaphragm, and correct breathing, 31, 65–71
Diarrhea, 44, 76

Diet, and dietary choices, 80–83, 153–55; and stress, 78–79, 81–82, 85
Digestion and digestive sequence, 21–26, 43–44, 76–79; dysfunction, 74–85; length of, 76, 129–30; and stress, 78–79
Digestive enzymes, 21, 33, 42–43
Dinan, Ted, quoted, 54–55
Distress, defined, 109
Dorsal motor nucleus, 13, 15
Drive-through car wash analogy, 75, 78
Drive-through effect, and digestion, 44
Dysautonomia, 102–103
Dysfunctions, 64–120; breathing, 31, 65–73; digestion, 74–85; and heart rate, 100–103; and liver, 104–107; and vagus nerve, 31, 64–120

Ears. *See* Auricular acupuncture
EECs (enteroendocrine cells), 89–90
Efferent neurons, 10–11
Electrical cord analogy, 58–59
Electrical stimulation, 163, 167–69
Electromagnetic frequencies (EMF), 126
Electronic devices, 138–39. *See also specific devices*
Emotional trauma. *See* Trauma
Endocrine pancreas, 23

Activate your VAGUS NERVE

HeartMath Inner Balance tool, 125, 150

Hepatic insulin sensitizing substance, 41

Herbicides, and food, 83–84

High blood pressure, 33. *See also* Blood pressure

Himalayan pink salt, 145

Hippocrates, quoted, 87

Hof, Wim. *See* Wim Hof Method

Holtz, Lou, quoted, 114

Hormones, 43; and blood pressure, 33. *See also specific hormones*

HRV. *See* Heart rate variability

Humming, 142–43

Hunger/satiety, 36–37, 76, 77, 84–85; and liver, 21, 22; and stress, 85

Hydration, nighttime, 139

Hydrochloric acid (HCl), 21

Hyman, Mark, 154

Hypochlorhydria (low stomach acid), 21

Hypothalamic-pituitary-adrenal (HPA) axis function, 113

Ileocecal valve, 78, 79–80

Immune activation, 93–99. *See also* Inflammation

Immune cells, and thymus, 18, 24, 45, 46, 47–51, 52, 87, 94–96

Immune system, 44–51; and stress, 49–51

Immunoglobulins, 47–48

In Defense of Food, 82

Infections, 46–47, 49–50

Inferior ganglion (nodose ganglion), 17

Inflammation, 11–12, 93–99; and trauma, 97–99; gut, 96–97; and stress, 4; and spleen, 24

Inner Balance tool from HeartMath, 125, 150

Insulin and insulin levels. *See* Blood sugar/insulin levels

Internet analogy, 10

Involution of thymus, 49

Jeffery, Ian B., quoted, 88

John, Elton, quoted, 153

Jugular foramen, 15, 16

Jugular ganglion (superior ganglion), 16

Keller, James, quoted, 170

Kharrazian, Datis, 160

Kidneys, 25; and blood pressure, 25, 32–33; and waste elimination, 34

Kondo, Marie, 139

Lactobacillus (Lacto) genus, 54–55

Laptops: and blue light exposure, 137–38; and posture, 70, 71

Large intestine, 25–26, 78–79, 86

Larynx: and breathing, 31, 70, 71, 72; and swallowing, 29, 77; and voice tone, 17, 19, 30

Laughter, 150–52

Leukocytes, 45, 47. *See also* White blood cells

Activate your VAGUS NERVE

Activate your VAGUS NERVE

GRATITUDE

This book could not have come to fruition if not for the support I have received from so many people.

First and foremost, Noureen, my rock: You have been beside me every step of the way and I don't think I can thank you enough for all you do. Writing this book has been a beautiful challenge, considering our life circumstances and our raising a beautiful daughter. You are the most supportive person I could ask for, and I thank you profusely for everything you have done and all that you will continue to do.

To my family: Mom, Dad, Afzal, and Faiz, you guys believed in me, and even though we were all in shock when I told you what was happening, you have been there behind me and I have felt your love throughout this journey. Thank you for always believing in me. Mummy, Papa, and Nida, thank you for encouraging me and keeping me looking forward always.

To my extended family, all my superfans: Thank you for all the words of encouragement and checking in on me to make sure our family was doing well through the process.

To Pedram: Thank you for talking to me at Mindshare, encouraging me to keep moving forward, and asking, "What have you done for me recently?" That question sparked an idea and allowed me to spread my wings.

To Bridget: Thank you for reaching out, believing in me, and supporting me on this journey. You have validated me and allowed me to believe in myself. Thank you.

And lastly, but certainly not least, to Team Proof. Sachin—who would've ever thought that since the day we met, you would inspire me to write this book, an accomplishment I had never even dreamed about until recently. Dipa, Ricky, Jared, Julie, Andrew, Carol, Jessica, Gillian, Gretchen, Marissa, Someya, Alice, Rachel, Sophia, and Angelito, thank you for the constant encouragement, support, and love. I am grateful for each one of you today and always.

Activate your VAGUS NERVE

ABOUT THE AUTHOR

Dr. Navaz Habib is a leading expert in the field of functional medicine and lifestyle interventions using vagus nerve activation. In overcoming his own health-related challenges, he has dedicated his career to addressing the root causes of inflammation, autoimmunity, and metabolic disorders, and improving the energy, focus, and motivation of his clients. Trained as a Doctor of Chiropractic and a Certified Functional Medicine Practitioner, Dr. Habib consults with high-performing entrepreneurs, executives, athletes, and professionals at his health clinic Health Upgraded and online through various courses and programs. Dr. Habib currently resides in Toronto, Canada, with his wife Noureen and their daughter Miraal.

Dr. Habib can be contacted through the following channels:

www.healthupgraded.com
www.drhabib.ca
Facebook: www.facebook.com/drnavazhabib
Instagram: @DrNavazHabib

Printed in the USA
CPSIA information can be obtained
at www.ICGtesting.com
CBHW050405250624
10599CB00010B/145

9 781612 438740